The Enigma of Advanced Nursing Practice

For my wife Anne and my parents
Lou and Les

The Enigma of Advanced Nursing Practice

Leslie P Woods

Quay Books

Mark Allen
Publishing Ltd

The enigma of advanced nursing practice

Quay Books Division, Mark Allen Publishing Ltd
Jesses Farm, Snow Hill, Dinton, Nr Salisbury, Wiltshire, SP3 5HN

British Library Cataloguing-in-Publication Data
A catalogue record is available for this book

© Mark Allen Publishing Ltd 2000
ISBN 1 85642 174 0

Printed in the UK by The Cromwell Press, Trowbridge, Wiltshire

Contents

List of Tables and Figures

Acknowledgements

My thanks are due to all the participants who took part in this study and willingly gave of their time, consideration and energy. I particularly owe a debt of gratitude to the five advanced nurse practitioners who were the main focus of the case studies, for without their help and tolerance, this study would not have been possible.

My thanks are also extended to my research supervisors, Professor John McLeod and Dr David Skidmore, whose critical comments, advice, guidance and words of support and encouragement were crucial to the development and completion of my PhD thesis.

I would like to extend my gratitude to the West Midlands NHS Executive who funded the Research Fellowship that allowed me to concentrate all of my energies on the task in hand.

Finally, I would like to thank my wife Anne for her unwavering support, patient understanding, incredible tolerance and continuing encouragement which were essential in helping me to maintain my sanity throughout the process.

Preface

It was Machiavelli who said, *'one change leaves the way open for the introduction of others'*. Undoubtedly, the sentiment of this statement will strike a familiar chord with the majority of nurses and healthcare workers in the UK. The seemingly constant state of change influencing the delivery of healthcare shows no sign of abating. Consequently, acknowledging that nursing is continually undergoing change, is somewhat self-evident (Frost, 1998). However, with any change comes opportunity. From a healthcare perspective, nurses in particular are increasingly finding themselves in positions whereby their skills and talents are in high demand and are at last being exploited to their full potential. There are many antecedents to the current trends in nursing practice development and role expansion. Some of the major catalysts that have shaped the way in which nursing has changed in recent years will be discussed in the *Introduction*. However, it is worthwhile mentioning here that the reconstruction of nursing practice is underpinned by two long-standing issues. The first concerns the pre-occupation nursing has with shaking off its image as a 'minor' profession (Retsas, 1995), while the second is associated with the needs driven ethos that prevails within the present day National Health Service (Salussolia, 1997). It has been suggested that:

> *'...the traditional concepts of nursing, together with the prescribed knowledge, values and skills, no longer seem to fit the experiences or desires of nurses who are increasingly being asked to identify their unique contribution to healthcare. Nurses are being faced with a conceptual and activity revision...'* (Graham, 1992, 118)

It needs to be acknowledged that practice development is by its nature fluid, dynamic and responsive to changing professional, social, political, and environmental factors. As such, nurses taking the lead in advancing practice need to be alert to having their skills and expertise exploited by other groups determined to follow their own agendas.

It was against a backdrop of political and professional change in the 1990s that a distinction between different levels of nursing practice and expertise is acknowledged to have emerged in the UK. In the debate that followed the United Kingdom Central Council for

Nursing, Midwifery and Health Visiting (UKCC) identification of the three levels of nursing practice (ie. professional, specialist and advanced practice) was polarised, with both supporters and opponents frequently courting controversy. While some in the profession sat back and waited to see the outcome of the debate, others used the initiative to educate and prepare nurses to take on new roles and responsibilities. Subsequently, an increasing number of nurses began the task of attempting to implement new roles in clinical practice. In the meantime, many in and outside the nursing profession struggled to come to terms with the concept of an advanced level of practice, and a state of confusion prevailed. Many looked to the UKCC, who had earlier agreed upon practice and educational criteria for the concept of a specialist level practitioner, to provide clarification for the concept of advanced practice. Little was forthcoming. Such was the level of disagreement and confusion about the notion of an advanced level of nurse practitioner, that in 1997 the UKCC announced that the term advanced practice was no longer appropriate. The reasons given for the U-turn were primarily related to the confusion the concept had created, coupled with the UKCC's own inability to reach consensus regarding relevant practice and educational criteria. Given the problems of definition and common understanding, the UKCC decided that it was necessary to replace the specialist practice framework it had originally hoped to develop (UKCC, 1998). In order to avoid the errors of the past, the UKCC set out on a consultation exercise in an attempt to arrive at a clear definition and agreed, generalisable practice standards of the concept that it now preferred to designate as *'a higher level of practice'* (UKCC, 1998). To the impartial observer, it appeared that the UKCC had introduced the concept of advanced practice, espoused its virtues, but then could not agree relevant practice criteria and standards, and, therefore, simply decided to ignore it. Little account was seemingly taken of those practitioners and organisations that had embraced the concept in the early to mid 1990s and had since taken steps to develop the idea by training and employing advanced practitioners. Consequently, to this day, the concept of advanced practice remains an enigma for many.

The purpose of this book is to add to the debate on advanced nursing practice that has gained momentum over recent years. It proposes a framework that will hopefully help nurses, managers, educationalists, physicians and, not least of all, advanced practitioners themselves to identify the key characteristics and traits of advanced practice. Despite innovative nursing roles beginning to emerge in the UK, little is known about the initial period of transition experienced by nurses who are required to reconstruct their practice to become advanced nurse practitioners (Brown & Olshansky, 1997). The purpose of this text is to enhance understanding of how nurses engage in the transitional process when moving from a position of experienced nurse to one of advanced nurse practitioner. The book will outline how the practises and attributes of advanced practitioners differ from those of their nursing colleagues. While various definitions and interpretations of advanced practice will be discussed, it is my position, perhaps somewhat controversially, that the pursuit of an ultimate definition of advanced practice is an erroneous endeavour. Those readers expecting to find such a definition at the conclusion of this book are warned that they will be disappointed.

The arguments put forward are taken from a study I conducted which examined the role transition of a small group of advanced nurse practitioners. As such, the discussion will draw not only on the theoretical and technical literature, but the evidence I collected over an intensive two-year period, along with my own ideas of the concept of advanced practice. Undoubtedly, some who read this text will disagree with its fundamental position. However, if this text can serve as an additional source of literature to stimulate debate, from which clarity and insight can be further derived, then it will have served its purpose. To simply ignore the concept of advanced practice in the hope it will go away both disregards the international context of the on-going development of nursing practice and does a disservice to those practitioners and organisations that have taken the risks associated with developing innovative practice developments.

References

Brown M, Olshansky E (1997) From limbo to legitimacy: a theoretical model of the transition to the primary care nurse practitioner role. *Nurs Research* **46**(1):46–51

Frost S (1998) Perspectives on advanced practice: an educationalist's view. In: Rolf G, Fulbrook P, eds. *Advanced Nursing Practice*. Butterworth-Heinemann, Oxford 33–42

Graham I (1992) Reconstructing nursing: a coronary care perspective of the primary nurse philosophy. *Inten Crit Care Nurs* **8**:118-124

Retsas A (1995) Knowledge and practice development: toward an ontology of nursing. *Aus J Adv Nurs* **12**(2):20–5

Salussolia M (1997) Is advanced nursing practice a post or a person? *Br J Nurs* **6**(16):928, 930–3

United Kingdom Central Council for Nursing, Midwifery and Health Visiting (1998) *A Higher Level of Practice: Consultation Document.* UKCC, London

Introduction

Why are you reading this book? On the face of it, a strange question for an author to ask his reader. Moreover, the question is one with a number of possible answers, ranging from simply being curious about the concept of advanced nursing practice, to having to prepare an academic assignment on the topic. There are, of course, many other reasons why you might be referring to this text. That you are reading this, however, a testament to the fact that the concept of an advanced level of nursing practice is worthy of further consideration and exploration. Before getting immersed in the main substance of the text, it is important to briefly review the antecedents that have led to the emergence of advanced nursing practice in the UK as a present day phenomenon.

Specialisation in nursing has been slow to evolve in the UK (Castledine,1991). However, this is a situation that has begun to change. In recent years, a number of strategic developments both within and outside the nursing profession have acted as catalysts for nurses to reflect on the nature of their clinical practice and consider ways in which it might be developed. While nurses and midwives have been expanding their clinical practice for many years (O'Flynn, 1996), recent debate has focused on the concept of different levels of practice and the expectation for nurses to develop new roles and working patterns (UKCC, 1993). The question this raises is, why has it taken so long for nurses to move on from simply extending their skills to advancing their practice in the broadest possible sense? This chapter attempts to provide an answer to this question by examining the background to the changes that have recently taken place in relation to the concept of advanced nursing practice. Rather than taking a historical look at the development of specific nursing roles in the UK, about which much has been previously written, this chapter will provide more of a global overview of the professional and political factors which, in my opinion, have had considerable impact on developments. I will argue that the convergence of three interrelated sets of conditions, occurring more or less simultaneously, either by design or coincidence, have given impetus to the drive for nurses to develop and advance their practice. These factors can be described as:

- the **desire** by, and for, nurses to develop and advance their practice

- the **recognition** for nurses to develop and advance their practice
- the **opportunity** for nurses to develop and advance their practice.

While these three conditions may have existed independently or in tandem in the past, it is conjectured that their simultaneous occurrence provides a basis for understanding the changes which have occurred in nursing practice and education in recent times. For the sake of clarity, each condition is discussed below. It should be acknowledged however, that many of the factors outlined in the following debate have had implications or impact on more than one condition.

The desire of and for nurses to advance their practice

It has been suggested that many nurses throughout the country would welcome the opportunity of expanding their roles (Cahill, 1996). This assertion is based not simply upon speculation, but on an increasing body of evidence which indicates that nurses have a genuine desire to advance their practice and to develop new roles (Last and Self, 1994; Barrett, 1995). Other professional groups, in particular medicine, are also eager that nurses should continue to develop their skills and abilities (Jewell and Turton, 1994; Barrett, 1995), although the motivation for their doing so has been questioned on grounds of exploitation (Giles, 1993).

The desire for nurses to advance their practice is also implicit in a number of national strategic documents to have appeared over the past decade including *A Vision for the Future* (DoH, 1993a) and *The Challenges for Nursing and Midwifery in the 21st century. The Heathrow Debate* (DoH,1993b). More recently, the policy document *Making a Difference* (DoH, 1999) has explicitly outlined the Government's desire to see nurses taking on more complex roles and having greater responsibility for the delivery of patient care. These documents explore the changing context of healthcare and outline strategic target areas where developments in nursing practice can be made. Albarran and Fulbrook (1998) make the point that in addition to strategies that explicitly address nursing, national priorities outlined in policy documents such as *The Health of the Nation* (DoH, 1992) have subsequently led to specialist nursing roles being forged to meet the needs of specific patient populations. This is one example where the opportunity for nurses to develop their practice can be linked to the desire to see the delivery of healthcare change. Likewise, the emergence of the concept of evidence-based practice, that is, the drive for increased clinical effectiveness and efficiency, also has implications for nurses to develop new roles (Kitson, 1997).

Consequently, the desire of and for nurses to advance their practice, while not being universally welcomed (Giles, 1993), is clearly evident. The UKCC has explicitly stated that it fully supports the notion of nurses advancing their practice (UKCC, 1997), even though it cannot agree upon the meaning of the concept of advanced practice. The most fundamental motive attached to the desire for nurses to advance their practice should not be overlooked in debates about efficiency and policy. It has been rightly acknowledged that patients or consumers are the group who should be the ultimate beneficiaries of nursing developments (Hunt and Wainwright, 1994). The benefits of nurse-led primary care clinics and nurse practitioners in accident and emergency departments provide just two of the many examples where changes to the way in which nursing care is delivered have met with the approval of patients as well as improving efficiency (Jones, 1994).

Nurses then appear to have the support from all quarters of the professional and public domains to advance their practice in new and novel ways. While the desire of and for nurses to advance their practice is evident in itself, it is insufficient to account fully for all the changes which have recently taken place.

Recognition for nurses to advance their practice

It is suggested that the second condition that has facilitated the process of nurses developing their practice revolves around the concept of recognition. In 1990, the UKCC's *Post Registration Education and Practice Project (PREPP)* report (UKCC, 1990) formally recognised three different levels of nursing practice. These were provisionally termed, 'primary', 'advanced' and 'consultant' practice. Differentiation between each level was provided in the form of a brief outline of the focus and scope of practice, as well as alluding to the level of educational preparation required. The UKCC later revised the titles corresponding to each level, preferring instead to call them 'professional', 'specialist' and 'advanced' practice respectively (UKCC, 1994), with the advanced level perceived as being highest and most complex.

While for some the notion of an advanced practitioner is not necessarily new (Mirr, 1993; Holyoake, 1995), it has been acknowledged that professional bodies in the UK have been slow to define and recognise the concept fully (Holyoake, 1995). Historically, the same can be said of other countries, where initially, advanced practice was not recognised as a discrete phenomenon (O'Flynn, 1996). Expectations that the concept of advanced practice would eventually be defined in the UK were raised when the PREPP report stated that the UKCC, at some later date, would produce specific details relating to the *'standard, kind and content of preparation for advanced practice'* (UKCC, 1990). Following the UKCC's revision of the nomenclature related to each level of practice however, this statement was found to refer to specialist practice and not advanced practice as initially anticipated.

The UKCC's precedent of acknowledging specialist and advanced levels of practice served to raise the expectations of nurses, managers and educationalists, and in effect legitimated the notion of nurses' advancing their practice to many both inside and outside the nursing profession. Furthermore, the concepts of specialist and advanced practice were perceived to provide nurses with a clinical career pathway which would enable them to be rewarded (financially) for remaining in clinical practice, as opposed to seeking promotion via traditional routes into education or management.

The concepts of specialist and advanced practice were given academic currency and recognition when the UKCC later confirmed that it expected the educational preparation of specialist practitioners to be at first degree level and advanced practitioners to be at the Master's degree level (UKCC, 1994). Thus, while the notion of specialist and advanced practitioners are not in themselves new ideas, the degree of recognition afforded these concepts, in particular by the UKCC, can be seen as a significant precursor to the developments that followed. Arguably, in formally recognising the concepts of specialist and advanced practice, the UKCC had provided an incentive for nurses to develop their practice and undertake further education and training. Moreover, it provided the impetus for universities to develop curricula that would provide the requisite educational programmes. In terms of healthcare providers, these developments allowed organisations to re-examine their service provision and explore ways in which specialist and advanced practitioners might be utilised in the delivery of healthcare in the future.

In addition to professional recognition, public recognition of the new roles and responsibilities anticipated of nurses in the future, is increasingly being made explicit in strategic policy documents, such as *Making a Difference* (DoH, 1999). Further acknowledgement of the way in which nursing roles are expected to develop was given high profile publicity in September 1998, when Prime Minister Tony

Blair announced that so-called 'consultant' nurses should be recognised for their experience and expertise in the delivery of healthcare. While this announcement was made in the context of problems with nurse recruitment, retention and career progress, it undoubtedly gave public recognition to the change in status of nursing. The inter-relationship, therefore, between the concept of recognition and the notion of desire of and for nurses to advance their practice, is clearly evident. While this combination strengthens the explanation for the drive of nurses to develop their practice base, the third condition perceived to have provided the final stimulus relates to the opportunity for nurses to advance their practice.

Opportunities for nurses to advance their practice

In the past, the opportunity for nurses to advance their practice was generally reliant upon locally agreed, ad hoc initiatives, which occurred sporadically in healthcare settings throughout the country. While these developments provided nurses with the opportunity to broaden their scope and sphere of practice, they remained relatively few in number and were often of short-term duration. It is suggested here that the current opportunity for nurses to advance their practice is based upon a series of recent events which are likely to lead to more widespread and sustainable developments in nursing practice.

The first of these events relates to a series of professional documents produced by the UKCC which outline the principles upon which any nurse can base their decision to develop and advance his or her practice. The key documents are perceived to be; the *Code of Professional Conduct* (UKCC, 1992a), *Exercising Accountability* (UKCC, 1989), and of particular importance, the *Scope of Professional Practice* (UKCC, 1992b). These documents clearly set out the UKCC's expectations with regard to the conduct and accountability of nurses, while at the same time opening the door to further development and expansion of clinical practice (Castledine, 1991). Arguably, the most liberating of the UKCC's documents is the *Scope of Professional Practice* (UKCC, 1992b) in which it is specifically stated that nurses are able to take on additional roles and responsibilities, providing they have the appropriate knowledge and training to do so. The *Scope of Professional Practice* (UKCC, 1992b) serves not only to recognise that nurses are increasingly in positions whereby they are likely to advance and develop their practice, but could also be interpreted as providing the momentum for the move toward independent nursing practice (Rieu, 1994). As such, the *Scope of Professional Practice* (UKCC, 1992b) has been seen as an instrument offering nursing endless opportunities (Autar, 1996).These professional documents, then, provide a clear framework for nurses to work from and as such allow them the opportunity of developing their practice while being free from the shibboleths that have held them back in the past.

The second factor providing nurses with the opportunity to advance their practice relates to changes in nurse education. The move toward nursing becoming an academic discipline as well as a practical one was signalled by the introduction of *Project 2000 (UKCC, 1986).* This not only led to changes in pre-registration programmes of education, but also provided the platform for the subsequent development of post-registration education and training and the integration of colleges of nursing and midwifery into the Higher Education sector. Since such mergers have taken place, there has been a proliferation of academically accredited post-registration nursing programmes at both the undergraduate and postgraduate levels. The UKCC's declaration that the academic preparation for specialist and advanced practitioners was expected to be at the first and Master's degree levels respectively, led a number of universities to design specific curricula aimed at preparing nurses to the requisite standard. As a result of such changes and new initiatives, nurses have seen a huge increase in the educational opportunities available to them in recent years.

The third, and perhaps most controversial, factor that has undoubtedly led to the opportunity for nurses to develop and advance their practice concerns changes to the working practices of junior doctors. The NHS Management Executive (1991) proposed a *New Deal* for junior doctors which involved a reduction in the number of hours they worked, while at the same time not increasing their number. This led healthcare trusts to confront the problem of how best they could meet the needs of the services they provided, while at the same time reducing the hours that junior medical staff worked. Inevitably, many trusts appeared keen to develop the route of nurses acting as partial substitutes for doctors (Cahill, 1996). The adoption of this strategy has led to the suspicion that the sole motive for trusts to employ nurses as specialist or advanced practitioners is for them to act primarily as replacements for junior doctors (Castledine, 1996). This argument is not new to nursing. Wright (1991) has already conceded that there is an established trend for nurses to extend their roles and take on doctors' duties.

An alternative view is that despite the potential for exploitation, a reduction in junior doctors' hours can be seen as sufficient reason for nurses to expand their roles (MacAlister and Chiam, 1995). Thus, in response to those critics who view the New Deal as being a strategy through which nurses can be exploited, there are those who consider that it legitimates the opportunity for nurses to develop their practice, while at the same time reducing junior doctor hours (Pickersgill, 1993).

These arguments draw attention to the contentious issue surrounding the difference between nurses **extending** their roles and **advancing** their practice. Extending practice, which has been the subject of a great deal of debate, is seen to be a task-oriented activity undertaken for the convenience of other professionals and at their discretion (Mitchinson and Goodlad, 1996). Extending roles on such a basis could be considered to be undesirable in the continuing quest for nursing to be recognised as a professional discipline in its own right. Advanced practice on the other hand, is seen by some to centre on the core therapeutic nursing roles of nurturing and caring and is focused on the delivery of holistic patient care (MacAlister and Chiam, 1995). Advancing practice on this basis is seen to be at the discretion of nursing and as such is viewed as being desirable professional development.

Interestingly, many of the concerns being expressed in the current debate were raised in the 1970s when there was a nation-wide shortage of doctors, and there were proposals that nurses might take over some of the doctors' clinical tasks and responsibilities (Castledine, 1991). The position of nursing, however, has significantly changed since the 1970s with regard to this whole issue. The UKCC have recognised that nurses are increasingly in positions whereby they can develop and advance their practice and have outlined a professional and educational framework to encourage them to do so. Furthermore, the desire of nurses themselves to advance their practice is evident from the many initiatives taking place nation-wide. These have seen nurses establish new roles such as nurse practitioners (Burgess, 1992); nurse anaesthetists (Carlisle, 1996); in nurse-led minor injury units (Beales and Baker, 1995); and even as a cardiac surgeon assistant (Holmes, 1994), to name but a few. While many of these developments can be linked to the political drive to reduce junior doctors' hours, they nonetheless serve to provide the opportunity, along with the desire and recognition, for nursing to develop and advance its own practice base.

It is the convergence of these three interrelated factors that may go some way toward explaining why you are reading this book. However, there are much more fundamental questions that you are likely to have on your mind such as, just what exactly is advanced practice? How is it recognised? And what differentiates the advanced practitioner from the experienced nurse? These are complex and difficult questions to answer and ones that have been asked of me many times. In the next chapter, I will focus on how the concept of advanced practice is explained and described in the literature, before going on and offering my own interpretation of this phenomenon in subsequent chapters.

References

Albarran J, Fulbrook P (1998) Advanced nursing practice: an historical perspective. In: Rolfe G, Fulbrook P, eds. *Advanced Nursing Practice.* Butterworth-Heinemann, Oxford:11–32

Autar R (1996) The scope of professional practice in specialist practice. *Br J Nurs* **5**(16):984–90

Barrett G (1995) To extend or not to extend — that is the question: A postal survey of opinions of nursing and medical staff regarding extended roles. *J Neonatal Nurs* **1** 3): 9–13

Beales J, Baker B (1995) Minor injuries units: expanding the scope of accident and emergency provision. *Acc Emerg Nurs* 3(2)65–7

Burgess K (1992) A dynamic role that improves the service: combining triage and nurse practitioner roles in A and E. *Prof Nurs* **7**(5):301–3

Cahill H (1996) Role definition: nurse practitioners or clinicians' assistants? *Br J Nurs* **5**(22):1382–6

Carlisle D (1996) Crossing the line. *Nurs Times* **92**(23):26–9

Castledine G (1991) The advanced nurse practitioner: part 1. *Nurs Stand* **5**(3):34–6

Castledine G (1996) The role and criteria of an advanced nurse practitioner. *Br J Nurs* **5**(5):288–9

Department of Health (1992) *The Health of the Nation: a Strategy for Health in England.* HMSO, London

Department of Health (1993a) *A Vision for the Future* HMSO, London

Department of Health (1993b) *The Challenges for Nursing and Midwifery in the 21st Century . The Heathrow Debate.* HMSO, London

Department of Health (1999) *Making a Difference.* HMSO, London

Giles S (1993) Passing the buck *Nurs Times* **89**(28):42–3

Holmes S (1994) Development of the cardiac surgeon assistant. *Br J Nurs* **3**(5):204–10

Holyoake D (1995) Advancing in Confusion *Nurs Stand* **9**(5):56

Hunt G, Wainwright P (1994) Introduction. In: Hunt G, Wainwright P eds. *Expanding the role of the nurse:The scope of professional practice.* Blackwell Scientific Publications, Oxford: x-xvi

Jewell D, Turton P (1994) What's happening to practice nursing? *Br Med J* **308**:735–6

Jones G (1994) Accident and emergency and the nurse practitioner. In: Hunt G, Wainwright P eds. *Expanding the role of the nurse:The scope of professional practice.* Blackwell Scientific Publications, Oxford: 162-181

Kitson A (1997) Using evidence to demonstrate the value of nursing. *Nurs Stand* **11**(28):34–9

Last T, Self N (1994) The expanded role of the nurse in intensive care. A national survey. In: Hunt G, Wainwright P, eds. *Expanding the Role of the Nurse: The Scope of Professional Practice.* Blackwell Scientific Publications, Oxford:114–31

MacAllister L, Chiam M (1995) Why do nurses agree to take on doctors' roles? *Br J Nurs* **4**(21):1238–9

Mirr M (1993) Advanced Clinical Practice: A Reconceptualized Role. *AACN* **4**(4):599–602

Mitchinson S, Goodlad S (1996) Changes in the roles and responsibilities of nurses. *Prof Nurs.* **11**(11):734–6

NHS Management Executive (1991) *Junior Doctors: The New Deal.* NHS Management Executive, London

O'Flynn A (1996) The preparation of advanced practice nurses. *Nurs Clin North Am* **31**(3):429–38

Pickersgill F (1993) A 'New Deal' for nurses too? *Nurs Stand* **7** (35):21–2

Rieu S (1994) Error and trial: the extended role dilemma. *Br J Nurs* **3** (4):168–74

United Kingdom Central Council for Nursing, Midwifery and Health Visiting (1986) *Project 2000. A New Preparation for Practice.* UKCC, London

United Kingdom Central Council for Nursing, Midwifery and Health Visiting (1989) *Exercising Accountability.* UKCC, London

United Kingdom Central Council for Nursing, Midwifery and Health Visiting (1990) *The Report of the Post-Registration and Education and Practice Project.* UKCC, London

United Kingdom Central Council for Nursing, Midwifery and Health Visiting (1992a) *Code of Professional Conduct for the Nurse, Midwife and Health Visitor.* UKCC, London

United Kingdom Central Council for Nursing, Midwifery and Health Visiting (1992b) *The Scope of Professional Practice.* UKCC, London

United Kingdom Central Council for Nursing, Midwifery and Health Visiting (1993) *Post-registration Education and Practice.* UKCC, London

United Kingdom Central Council for Nursing, Midwifery and Health Visiting (1994) *The Future of Professional Practice – The Council's Standards for Education and Practice Following Registration.* UKCC, London

United Kingdom Central Council for Nursing, Midwifery and Health Visiting (1997) *The Council's Decision on PREP and Advanced Practice Registrar's Letter 8/1997. UKCC, London*

Wright S (1991) Nursing Development. *Nurs Stand* **5**(38):52–3

I

Deconstructing the concept of advanced practice

While acknowledging that the notion of advancing nursing practice appears to be a generally welcomed concept in the UK, the absence of an agreed definition of advanced practice and the failure to recognise advanced practitioners have proven problematic. In other countries, such as Australia, Canada and the USA, these concepts have become widely accepted over the past 30 years and during that time a substantial body of literature has evolved relating to the many facets of advanced nursing practice. In the UK, however, there is a dearth of empirical data and literature regarding this field of study, given the relatively early stage in the development of advanced nurse practitioners (ANPs) in this country. This is a situation which is gradually beginning to change, but does mean that any review of the literature regarding the concept of advanced practice inevitably draws on the body of international literature that has developed over the past three decades. As a result, account needs to be taken of the trans-cultural nature of the literature and the degree that one can transfer constructs and interpretations to a UK context.

Definitions of advanced practice and advanced practitioners

Arriving at a definition of the term 'advanced practice' is problematic (Patterson and Haddad, 1992; Davies and Hughes, 1995; Woods, 1997). One of the main reasons why this is so is because the nature of nursing practice, especially that considered to be advanced, varies greatly between the different clinical contexts and settings. As a result, definitions of advanced practice have remained largely non-specific and broad in scope. The rationale for this strategy appears to be the belief that imprecise definitions help to facilitate creativity and innovation in clinical practice (Mirr, 1993). The UKCC's (1994b) initial attempt at a definition of an advanced practitioner can be seen to have followed this trend, when it stated that the advanced nurse practitioner will:

> *'...be concerned with adjusting the boundaries for the development of future practice, pioneering and developing new roles responsive to changing needs and, with advancing*

clinical practice, research and education to enrich professional practice as a whole.' (p5)

The use of the terms 'adjusting the boundaries', 'pioneering and developing new roles' and 'to enrich professional practice as a whole', all indicate a lack of specificity to the definition, appearing to place the responsibility on individual practitioners to be creative in developing their practice.

Another UK writer offers a personal view of what he believes to be the definition of advanced nurse practitioners. He states they should be:

'...specially prepared nurses who are working in roles which demand a lot of nursing experience, education at master's degree level, and nursing skills that contribute to meeting the complex needs of vulnerable people and the need to be continuously questioning the fundamentals and boundaries of nursing.' (Castledine, 1996, p288)

The definition is augmented by a list of seven categories which are proposed should form the criteria, roles and functions of advanced nurse practitioners in the UK. The categories can be seen to serve the purpose of adding a degree of specificity to an otherwise general definition. The key criteria listed for the advanced practitioner are that they should be: an autonomous practitioner; experienced and knowledgeable; a researcher and evaluator of care; expert in health and nursing assessment; expert in case management; a consultant, educator and leader; and respected and recognised by others in the profession. This list tends to focus on a series of roles that advanced practitioners are expected to perform, while at the same time elaborating on some of the attributes required of an advanced practitioner. However, with the exception of mentioning health and nursing assessment, the criteria stop short of identifying specific nursing practices. The trend for defining the concept of advanced practice in terms of a series of roles appears to be commonplace in the nursing literature (Sparacino and Cooper, 1990; Pickler and Reyna, 1996). Moreover, this approach continues to prevail, as is evident in the early attempts to define the nature of the new 'nurse consultant' posts in the UK (NHS Executive, 1999).

Some definitions of advanced practice do not, however, limit themselves to conveying the concept of advanced practice as simply a series of roles. One of the most comprehensive and recent definitions of advanced practice is offered by the American Nurses' Association Congress of Nursing Practice, which states that:

'Nurses in advanced clinical nursing practice have a graduate degree in nursing. They conduct comprehensive health assessments and demonstrate a high level of autonomy and expert skill in the diagnosis and treatment of complex responses of individuals, families and communities to actual or potential health problems. They formulate clinical decisions to manage acute and chronic illness and promote wellness. Nurses in advanced clinical practice integrate education, research, management, leadership and consultation into their clinical role. They function in collegial relationships with nursing peers, physicians, professionals, and others who influence the health environment'. (McLoughlin, 1992. p23)

This definition identifies several features which are viewed as being nursing-focused (Mirr, 1993) and essential characteristics of advanced practice and advanced practitioners. These include:

- graduate education
- expert and skilled clinicians, with the ability to not only care for, but to diagnose and treat complex conditions
- autonomous practitioners, with the ability to formulate clinical decisions based on their clinical judgement
- a health, as well as disease focus to the care they provide in their clinical role
- the integration of the sub-roles of educator, researcher, manager, leader, and consultant into an eclectic clinical role
- an ability to function in multidisciplinary and collegiate relationships with other professionals in the healthcare environment.

While some may consider this definition and its characteristics to be comprehensive in nature, critics may claim it to be somewhat Utopian and concede that only in exceptional circumstances would a nurse be able to fulfil all of these requirements to maximum effect. The problems inherent in attempting to define such a complex phenomenon as advanced practice in isolation have led to a number of definitions, especially from the USA, to describe advanced practice in relation to specific practice models such as nurse practitioners and clinical nurse specialists.

To date, most definitions of advanced practice and advanced practitioners have focused on either the specific roles such nurses undertake, or the tasks they perform. While a number acknowledge that the level of academic preparation expected to become an advanced practitioner is at a Master's degree level, they fail to elaborate on the cognitive characteristics required to become a competent practitioner. Smith (1996), however, tends to emphasise the cognitive attributes above others when she states that:

> *'The advanced practice nurse in the Australian context is an independent nurse practitioner who uses expert problem solving skills that are a result of complex reasoning, critical thinking, and analysis to form clinical judgements. Hence, nursing practice is less likely to be a task behaviour, and practice is embedded in theory and research. The advanced practice nurse's activities are not limited to the physical and psychosocial aspects of an individual's care but ... incorporate education, research, and the contribution to health policy formulation.'* (p552)

In this definition, complex reasoning and problem solving skills are tied not only into patient care activities, but also into other activities as diverse as education and health policy formulation. Smith (1996) goes on to argue that viewing nursing practice in terms of task behaviour is unhelpful when trying to conceptualise the complexity of advanced practice. Davies and Hughes (1995) too, consider that any attempt to deconstruct the advanced practice role into its component parts is unhelpful. They assert that the essence of advanced nursing practice is more a 'way of thinking' or a 'world view based on knowledge', rather than simply a series of roles. In the UK, Manley (1996) lends her support to the argument that the complexity of advanced practice cannot be developed or even recognised from a behaviourally-based checklist of standards. The UKCC echoed this sentiment when they arrived at a similar conclusion following the consultation exercise regarding the definition of advanced practice. They claimed that there was:

> *'...widespread agreement that advanced practice was not about tasks but a broader concept of nursing, midwifery and health visiting and particularly about advancing the practice of others. It was felt that a checklist of standards would conflict with the dynamic and autonomous nature of the concept of advancing practice.'* (UKCC, 1997b)

The definition of the concept of advanced practice is clearly equivocal. A number the definitions do share, either explicitly or implicitly, certain characteristics which appear to be central to the notion of advanced practice. These can be summarised as comprising:

- graduate education and preparation
- possession of expert clinical and cognitive skills
- an expert clinician, who is both knowledgeable and experienced
- independence and autonomy in the organisation of clinical practice
- role eclecticism; including the sub-roles of clinician, educator, researcher, administrator, innovator and consultant
- ability to function in collegiate relationships with other healthcare providers
- a world view of advanced nursing practice which guides thinking.

Which, if any, of these characteristics takes precedence, or how they are incorporated into the delivery of nursing care, depends upon the model of advanced practice adopted.

Arriving at a globally accepted definition of advanced practice then is clearly polemic, if not impossible, as any such statement would primarily serve to rigidify the concept and could potentially inhibit innovation. In the absence of such a definition, it appears logical that the notion of advanced practice is best understood and debated in terms of the series of personal and practice characteristics and attributes demonstrated by advanced practitioners.

Attributes and characteristics of advanced practitioners

While the attributes and characteristics of advanced practitioners have been alluded to in the previous discussion, they generally receive little attention in the literature (Patterson and Haddad, 1992). An overview of the limited literature highlights a number of desirable characteristics and attributes in the cognitive, affective and behavioural domains of the individual, as well as emphasising the importance of the personal and professional experience of the practitioner. Examples of four such characteristics are briefly discussed below: leadership, clinical judgement and decision-making; personal qualities; cognition and knowledge base.

Leadership

Spross and Baggerly (1989) reviewed and critiqued a number of conceptual models and frameworks of clinical nurse specialist practice and believe one of the essential attributes of the advanced practitioner to be that of effective leadership. This is not surprising as the concept of leadership is common to a number of models and definitions of advanced practice, including the new nurse consultant posts in the UK (Holt, 1984; McLoughlin, 1992; Ackerman *et al*, 1996; Pickler and Reyna, 1996; Manley, 1997; Goodman, 1998, NHS Executive, 1999). Patterson and Haddad (1992) emphasise that one of the properties of leadership is that it exists on more than one plane. At the higher level, they see advanced practitioners as a major force in moving the nursing profession forward as a whole, whereas at a lower level (but of equal importance), they see advanced practitioners being able to demonstrate the use of theory-based practice to other nurses. The latter is seen as a way of establishing ANPs as clinically based leaders (Sutton and Smith, 1995). This interpretation of leadership appears to have been used by the UKCC (1994c) as one way of differentiating between specialist and advanced practice. In the case of the specialist practitioner, the UKCC anticipate that leadership will focus predominantly on clinical practice and in particular, the monitoring and improvement of standards of care at a local level. Advanced practice on the other hand, is said to be concerned with not only advancing clinical practice, but also enriching professional practice as a whole, ie. at a higher level. Therefore, there appears to be a considerable degree of consensus that one of the essential attributes of an advanced practitioner is that of leadership.

Clinical judgement and decision-making

The second attribute to receive attention in the literature relates to the concept of clinical judgement and decision making. Expertise in decision-making is perceived to be one of the distinctive attributes of the advanced practitioner (Snyder and Yen, 1995). While the terms clinical judgement and decision-making are sometimes used interchangeably, they can in fact be viewed as distinct entities. Clinical judgement concerns the ability to make distinctions between different conditions and situations, whereas decision-making is the process of arriving at an appropriate course of action based upon one's clinical judgement. In this way, it is acknowledged that one informs the other and that in the case of advanced practitioners, autonomous decision-making is validated by advanced clinical judgement (Joynes, 1996).

Spross and Baggerly (1989) describe decision-making as a complex intellectual process which others have argued is influenced by the two essential factors of knowledge and experience (Watson, 1994). Clinical judgement and decision-making are consequently seen to be reliant upon:

> *'...the interaction and integration of graduate education in nursing practice [providing the knowledge] and years of clinical experience.'* (Spross and Baggerly, 1989, p20)

It is believed that this combination enables advanced practitioners to exercise clinical judgement at an advanced level (Snyder and Yen, 1995). Interestingly, the UKCC's (1994a) expectation of the specialist practitioner, not only the advanced practitioner, is to possess the ability to make clinical judgements at a higher level, although the educational preparation required for such is only considered to be necessary at the first degree level. The absence of studies comparing the clinical judgement of advanced (USA and UK) and specialist (UK only) practitioners, prevents the qualitative differences between the two groups being elicited.

Personal qualities

Unlike decision-making and leadership, which to some degree can be considered to be observable behaviours and learned attributes, the affective characteristics inherent in the individual can neither be easily learned nor observed. Yet these attributes are seen to be of importance in distinguishing advanced practitioners from other nurses. Patterson and Haddad (1992) list a number of such attributes including: being a risk taker and willing to 'bend' the rules (Sutton and Smith, 1995); being a visionary to utilise and guide nursing research; having an inquiring mind to participate in research; being flexible and open to new ideas. In addition, it has been suggested that advanced practitioners value the uncertainty generated in practice situations by identifying it as an opportunity for growth and further development (Sutton and Smith, 1995). Whether each of these attributes is present in all advanced practitioners is difficult to confirm.

Cognition and knowledge base

O'Rourke (1989) emphasises the cognitive attributes of advanced practitioners, which are implicit in some of the characteristics previously discussed. She suggests that advanced practitioners have the capacity to self-direct; modify theory to practice implementation; re-perceive knowledge and/or re-arrange it to develop new theory; transfer knowledge; introduce new learning. For some, these attributes characterise the notion of critical reflection (Sutton and Smith, 1995), along with competence in critical thinking and analysis, which are considered to be the essential characteristics of advanced nursing practice (Davies and Hughes, 1995). It is attributes such as these which underpin the belief in the importance of graduate education, which is seen to be significant in providing a comprehensive knowledge base for advanced practitioners in their practice (Calkin, 1984; King *et al*, 1996). A highly developed knowledge base and the cognitive capacity of deliberate reasoning, combined with intuition and experience, enables advanced practitioners to perceive situations in new ways and to develop their clinical practice accordingly (Calkin, 1984; Joynes, 1996).

Arguably, many of these personal characteristics and attributes are present to some degree in the majority of nurses, yet not all nurses are perceived to be, or perceive themselves to be, advanced practitioners. Patterson and Haddad (1992) account for this difference when they argue:

> *'While countless numbers of nurses may be well developed in one or more of these attributes, it is not until all are present in combination that the nurse may be clearly identified as one who is practicing at an advanced level; who is continuously growing and developing professionally; and who is leading and contributing to the growth and improvement of nursing.'* (p19)

The attributes and characteristics of the practitioner clearly underpin the concept of advance practice, regardless of the operational or conceptual model adopted, or the environment in which practice occurs. Arguably, such attributes are as important as the roles that advanced practitioners are expected to perform, or the skills they possess. However, they are far more difficult to observe, measure or quantify. Consequently, the literature tends to be dominated by the roles and functions advanced practitioners carry out, with the result that various operational and conceptual models have evolved over recent years.

Models of advanced practice

A variety of roles and practice models have been developed within the nursing profession, all of which claim to be forms of advanced practice (Patterson and Haddad, 1992). The practice model adopted by a practitioner is determined by a multiplicity of factors including: the nature of the clinical environment; the needs of the patient/client group; deployment and organisational goals; the preparation of the advanced practitioner; local and national regulations governing nursing practice; and, not least of all the philosophy of the individual practitioner. This results in variations in the way in which advanced roles are operationalised (Russell and Hezel, 1994) with the consequence that a number of differences both within and between categories of advanced practitioners are evident (Patterson and Haddad, 1992).

Traditionally, advanced practitioners have been differentiated by the roles and functions they perform, and the setting in which practice takes place (Pickler and Reyna, 1996). In the USA, the term *advanced practice* describes four categories of practitioner (Uckan *et al* 1994); Nurse Practitioners (NP); Clinical Nurse Specialists (CNS): Certified Registered Nurse Anaesthetists; and Certified Nurse Midwives (Mirr, 1993; Bachus, 1995). In the context of this discussion, these are referred to as **operational** models[1] In addition to the operational models, a number of **conceptual** models of advanced practice have been posited in an attempt to explain the unique characteristics of advanced nursing practice. These models are abstractions and attempt to locate the construct of advanced practice into a variety of conceptual frameworks. Given the focus of this book and its length, there is insufficient space to consider the merits and limits of the various conceptual models that have been developed over the years. For the meantime, attention will be given to the two dominant operational models of advanced practice, the nurse practitioner and the clinical nurse specialist.

The nurse practitioner model

The nurse practitioner role is considered to have developed as a result of a collaborative venture between nurses and physicians responding to changes in the US healthcare delivery system and a maldistribution of providers in the late 1960s (Fenton and Brykczynski, 1993). The main role was perceived to be one of a provider of patient care (Ford and Silver, 1967) with nurse practitioners being traditionally employed in primary or ambulatory care settings in the USA (Mirr, 1993). Educational programmes to prepare nurses to become nurse practitioners took a life course

---

1   The review will not include literature pertaining to Certified Registered Nurse Anaesthetists or Certified Nurse Midwives, as both these unique roles are peripheral to the focus of this text.

focus, as opposed to a disease or discipline focus. Consequently, nurses were prepared as either paediatric nurse practitioners, adult nurse practitioners, family nurse practitioners and more recently, gerontological nurse practitioners.

The delivery of healthcare has, however, changed rapidly in recent years (Watts *et al*, 1996) and has resulted in the movement of nurse practitioners into acute care settings (Keane *et al*, 1994). Amongst the reasons cited for the shift toward acute care nurse practitioners is the:

'...response to social and financial pressures, anticipated residency shortages, and an anticipated decrease in existing barriers to practice.' (Keane *et al*, 1994, p232)

Arguably, a number of these factors are reflected in the UK healthcare system and account, at least in part, for the movement toward the expansion of nurses' roles and responsibilities in this country.

The demand for nurse practitioners was such that a proliferation of certificate level and continuing education programmes were developed (NONPF, 1990). A particular problem with these courses was that they varied both in level and duration (Kitzman, 1989). However, the number of non-degree courses has been on the decrease in recent years, and correspondingly, the number of Master's degree courses is on the increase (NONPF, 1990).

The nurse practitioner role has traditionally had a uni-dimensional focus, primarily concerned with the direct delivery of patient care (Kitzman, 1989). Practice has been identified as including; physical and psychosocial assessment; history taking; physical examination; ordering and interpreting diagnostic investigations; and developing and implementing therapeutic interventions in collaboration with other healthcare providers (Ford, 1979). Nurse practitioners are generally afforded prescriptive privileges in the USA, although there is considerable variation to the limitations of prescriptive authority from state to state (Pearson, 1995). To summarise:

'Nurse practitioners provide primary healthcare services to clients - individuals, families, and groups - emphasizing the promotion of health and the prevention of disease. They manage actual and potential health problems, which include common diseases and human response to disease. Consultation and referral occur as needed...' (American Nurses' Association, 1987, p2)

The nurse practitioner is increasingly prepared at the Master's degree level and is perceived to possess advanced clinical skills and reasoning, as well as being afforded prescriptive privileges.

The nurse practioner model in the UK

The ability to make comparisons between nurse practitioners in the UK and those in the USA is limited. The UKCC (1997a) considers that the majority of nurse practitioner graduates in the UK fulfil the requirements for the specialist level of practice. Nurse prctitioners on the other hand, consider that acceptance and development of their roles, have been impeded by a lack of professional recognition from the UKCC (Torn and McNicol, 1998). This is due in part to the notion that the nurse practitioner role is considered to consist of nurses taking on technical or medically related tasks and procedures (Castledine, 1994). The UKCC's decision is also likely to be influenced by the level of academic preparation of nurse practitioners, which has been shown to be inconsistent in terms of both academic level and duration. This is illustrated by the preparation to become a nurse practitioner ranging from a few study days (Howie, 1992; Jones 1994) to a four month training programme (Burgoyne, 1992), and in one instance a 2 year part-time diploma programme (Simon, 1992). To meet the criteria for advanced practitioners initially laid down by the UKCC, the level of academic preparation would be expected to be at least Master's degree level, which the above clearly fail to achieve, although increasingly there appears to be a shift toward graduate preparation.

Further variance in the standard of preparation and orientation of nurse practitioner practice can be explained by the way in which the development of such posts has tended to be in response to local initiatives, as opposed to a national strategy or training programme. As a result, nurse practitioners are deployed sporadically throughout all levels of the healthcare system and work in a variety of contexts, including for example; in primary care with General Practitioners (Stilwell *et al,* 1987); in accident and emergency departments (Howie, 1992; Burgoyne 1992; Jones, 1994) and in nurse practitioner led clinics (Hill, 1992). While nurse practitioners undertake activities and perform skills not possessed by other nurses, their scope and sphere of practice may appear limited when compared to many of their US counterparts. One exception to this rule appears to be in the emergence of advanced neonatal nurse practitioners, whose role appears to be similar to that of their counterparts in the US (Doherty, 1996; Dillon and George, 1997).

While variations in the context and practices of nurse practitioners inevitably exist in the US, there remains a general consensus with regard to the expectations of the level of preparation and clinical practice. In addition, in the US each state has its own regulatory procedure and strict accreditation system which determines the scope of practice of advanced practice nurses (Pearson, 1995). A similar framework is not currently in existence in the UK and consequently there is a huge variation in the preparation and practice of nurse practitioners. Work has recently been conducted to identify and map the competencies and parameters of the nurse practitioner role (Roberts-Davis *et al*, 1998) so that a clearer picture of nursing development in this area can be assessed. Similarly, the UKCC is exploring ways in which recognition as a higher level practitioner can be regulated (UKCC, 1998).

The clinical nurse specialist model

The development of the CNS role is said to be largely attributed to the rapid progress made in medical technology in 1960s and the subsequent need for specialised and complex nursing care (Menard, 1987). The development of CNS practice has, therefore, taken place predominantly within hospital settings (Mirr, 1993). The primary purpose of the CNS role was seen as being the improvement of patient care (Crabtree, 1979; Holt, 1984). The title of 'clinical nurse specialist' in the UK, however, was not in common usage until the late 1980s (Manley, 1997) and even then roles were notably different in their orientation, scope and preparation (Manley, 1993). As in the US, the development of the CNS role in the UK has been linked to the technological explosion in healthcare and has resulted in a plethora of different titles. In most cases, specialisation appears to reflect an associated medical discipline (Pickersgill, 1995) as opposed to a life course focus, such as, clinical nurse specialist in epilepsy, clinical nurse specialist in diabetes and so on. Whereas in the US, the CNS is acknowledged as an advanced practitioner, the UKCC considers the majority of its UK counterparts to be practising at a specialist, rather than advanced, level of practice (UKCC, 1997a).

In the US, only clinical nurse specialists are **required** to possess a Master's degree in order to practice (American Nurses' Association, 1986). In the UK, while some CNSs possess Master's degrees, the usual route to achieving status as a clinical nurse specialist has been via the accumulation of knowledge and experience over an extended period of time. There are few, if any, university programmes specifically designed to prepare clinical nurse specialists and consequently there is widespread variance in the level of type of preparation in the UK (Woods, 1997).

The CNS role is widely acknowledged as being multidimensional and multifaceted (Kitzman, 1989).

'The clinical nurse specialist ... is an expert in clinical practice, an educator, a consultant, a researcher, and administrator...'
(American Nurses' Association, 1986, p2)

However, while providing some direct care, the CNS spends more time in consultation, education and administration (Kitzman, 1989) and less on research (Cooper and Sparacino, 1990), despite expert practice being originally conceived as the pivotal role (Keane *et al*, 1994). In stark contrast to nurse practitioners, clinical nurse specialists have generally been denied prescriptive authority privileges in the majority of states in the US. Wolf (1990) asserts that over time the CNS role has been diverted from its original purpose, ie. that of providing specialised nursing care and that administrators have deployed their expertise in order to meet broader institutional needs. Furthermore, Hamric (1989) asserts that some nurses use the title of CNS as a mark of educational or clinical prestige, rather than a title that describes their role function.

To summarise, the clinical nurse specialist model of practice has a wider scope of practice in terms of education, consultation, research, administration and policy development, as well as the delivery of direct patient care. CNSs generally practice in secondary and tertiary care settings in the US, while in the UK, some practice in primary care. The CNS must be prepared at the Master's degree level in the US, but not so in the UK. CNSs work in collaborative relationships with other healthcare workers and administrators, but are not afforded the prescriptive privileges given to nurse practitioners.

The clinical nurse specialist and nurse practitioner roles were conceived to meet different aims and objectives, yet in recent years there has been increasing debate in the US regarding the merits of merging the two roles into one advanced practice role (Page and Arena, 1994). The premise underpinning this idea is that the uniqueness of each role has blurred over time (Pickler and Reyna, 1996). Disagreements with regard to the direction, desirability and feasibility of such a merger are commonplace (Hanson and Martin, 1990). While the two roles have claims to distinct functions, it is also claimed that many of their facets can be effectively interfaced (Ditzenberger *et al*, 1995). Mirr (1993) argues, however, that the evolution of these two roles should not be considered as one moving into the setting of the other:

'... but, rather, an advanced practice role that uses multiple practice models and a variety of settings.' (pp599-600)

It has been suggested that as roles begin to merge, practitioners will be known as Advanced Practice Nurses (Monicken, 1995) and evidence exists to suggest that this change in nomenclature has already begun to take place (Uckan *et al*, 1994).

While there are some differences in emphasis between the various operational models of advanced practice which are becoming increasingly commonplace, there are many similarities. Two operational models appear to dominate, the CNS model, with a prominent focus on the *system* of care and care provision and, the NP model, with a prominent focus on the *recipient* of care and care delivery. The eclectic clinical nurse specialist/nurse practitioner model, which some claim has equal focus on the system and delivery of care, is difficult to reconcile. The writers who claim this model of practice to be effective (see: Hunsberger *et al,*1992; Ditzenberger *et al,* 1995; Ackerman *et al,* 1996) have a tendency to describe role dualism as opposed to role eclecticism. They envisage the practitioner acting in **either** a CNS type role or a nurse practitioner capacity at different times. Consequently, they appear to have in effect failed to achieve an integrative model of practice to which they originally aspired. That is not to say that such an eclectic model of practice is not possible, rather, it is a case that to date the evidence of the development of such a role remains unconvincing.

As for the other models of practice, such as the nurse consultant model outlined by a number of writers (Wright, 1994; Mills, 1996; Smith, 1996; Manley, 1997), the role as described shares so many similarities with the CNS model of practice that the two could be subsumed into one role. Likewise, the nurse clinician model as described by Gibbon and Luker (1995) for example, shares so many similarities with the NP that the two accounts are virtually describing the same role. It remains to be seen whether the new nurse consultant role advocated for the UK becomes unique and discernible in its own right. The four core functions anticipated of the new consultant nurse posts: expert practice; professional leadership and consultancy; education, training and development; and practice and service development, research and evaluation (NHS Executive, 1999) share many features and characteristics common to both the NP and CNS models described earlier. At this time however, it appears that the specification for the new post leans toward the CNS model of practice, rather than that of the NP model, although only time will reveal if this will be the case. Whatever the outcome, one might argue that adding more titles and different nomenclature to what are ostensibly very similar advanced practice roles, simply muddies the water and adds to the confusion already surrounding the subject.

Nursing versus the medical model of advanced practice

Any discussion of models of advanced practice cannot be complete without reference to the arguments that prevail as to which practice paradigm advanced practitioners belong, nursing or medicine. In the UK, this argument has been fuelled by the prospect of nurses' expanding their roles into activities that were once the prerogative of doctors. The predictable result is that nurses have been accused of becoming doctor substitutes or 'mini-doctors' (Castledine, 1995; Mathieson 1996). Consequently, their identity has been more closely associated with that of medical practitioners, as opposed to nurses. Recent developments, such as the role of nurse surgical assistant (Tuthill, 1995), whose explicit objective is to provide assistance to the surgeon with the aim of reducing the number of junior doctors' hours, clearly provides the foundation for such an argument.

In examining the practice of advanced practitioners, there is clearly evidence that nurses are able to undertake many of the activities, traditionally viewed within the realm of medicine, and perform them with equal competence. Both in the US and the UK, studies have been undertaken which compare the effectiveness of nurse practitioners with that of doctors (Spitzer *et al,* 1974; Sox, 1979; Salkever *et al,* 1982; United States Congress, Office of Technology Assessment, 1986; Greenhalgh and Co Ltd, 1994; Touche Ross Management Consultants, 1995). It can be argued, that while such studies attempt to demonstrate that the practice capabilities of nurse practitioners compare favourably with those of medical practitioners, an inevitable consequence of such inquiries is to locate the concept of advanced nursing practice within the medical paradigm. Smith (1995) argues that in the US, advanced nursing practice has been nurtured by the medical model and in the process is at risk of being defined by the medical model, in terms of:

'...an expanded knowledge base to support diagnosis, prevention, and treatment of disease.' (Smith, 1995, p2)

She argues that in so doing, advanced practice nurses define themselves as physician assistants or as a physician extension, as opposed to filling the identified gap in healthcare with a core of nursing practice.

The argument then, as to whether advanced nursing practice is located within a medical or nursing paradigm, is often a sophistry, as the real debate is founded on the medicalised tasks that such nurses are perceived to perform. Consequently, some advanced practice nurses, in particularly nurse practitioners, whose role has a uni-dimensional focus and who are seen to be able to perform procedures and tasks associated with medical practice, are more likely to be labelled as practising from a medical model. It is often this aspect of the NP role that is overemphasised (Casey, 1995). Alternatively, clinical nurse specialists, whose role has a multi-dimensional focus involving the patient, nursing staff, and the organisation, are more likely to be seen to be practising from a nursing model. Advanced practice nurses themselves, whether they be CNSs or NPs, would argue that they practice primarily from a nursing paradigm (Garland and Marchione, 1982; Thibodeau and Hawkins, 1994), but are able to incorporate medical tasks and procedures into their work with patients when required and where permitted.

Upon closer scrutiny, the nursing versus medical model debate, primarily revolves around two issues: the deployment of nurses to provide a service (or part thereof) previously provided by another healthcare worker, usually a doctor; and the performance of procedures and tasks predominantly associated as having a medical orientation. This has led to what Thibodeau and Hawkins (1994) call *'role parallelism'*, whereby some practitioners imitate a medical ethos and physician behaviours in order to boost their role confidence. However, Thibodeau and Hawkins (1994) concluded from their study involving 482 nurse practitioners, that:

> *'...nurse practitioners...see themselves as nurses with a broader focus than that inherent in the medical paradigm.'*
> (p215)

It appears that advanced practice nurses predominantly see themselves functioning within a nursing framework (Snyder and Yen, 1995). It is argued, however, that some practitioners fail to explain the specialist nursing knowledge they possess in relation to their field of practice in favour of emphasising the skills and knowledge they have gained from medicine (Chickadonz and Perry, 1985). It is this trait that appears to label advanced nursing practice as originating from a 'medical model'.

The real debate then has little to do with the foundation of a philosophical basis for guiding nursing practice and more to do with how clinical practice is organised, along with the additional skills that some nurses possess. The argument of advanced practitioners practising from either a nursing or medical model is therefore spurious and misleading and serves only to cloud our present understanding of advanced nursing practice (Bajnok, 1988).

Conclusion

Reviewing the literature reveals that while arriving at a global definition of advanced practice is problematic, the essential characteristics of the concept can be extracted from the varying interpretations of the construct which have been developed. To date, attempts at describing advanced practice and even developing conceptual models of advanced practice have generally relied on the identification of a series of roles and task behaviours to explain the phenomenon. The majority of such models, perhaps with the exception of Benner (1984), remain to have their validity established.

In addition to the conceptual models of advanced practice that have been developed over recent years, a number of operational models have been identified. It has been asserted above that, while various operational models exist, most could be subsumed under two principal models of advanced practice, namely the nurse practitioner or the clinical nurse specialist. Arguably, the personal attributes of the practitioner, rather than their title or the identification of a series of skills they are able to perform, capture the essence of advanced practice. It is not only that these attributes and characteristics are present in advanced practitioners, but that they are developed to an expert degree to allow their practice to be differentiated from that of their colleagues. The concept of expertise and that of the expert practitioner will be taken up in the next chapter.

References

Ackerman M, Norsen L, Martin B *et al* (1996) Development of a model of advanced practice *Am J Crit Care* **5**(1):68–73

American Nurses' Association. (1986) *The role of the clinical nurse specialist.* Publication No. NP-70 2M. American Nurses' Association, Kansas

American Nurses' Association. (1987) *Standards of practice for the primary healthcare nurse practitioner.* Publication No. NP-70 2M. American Nurses' Association, Kansas

Bachus K (1995) Advanced registered nurse practitioners: preparation, roles and practice settings. *Kansas Nurs* **70**(9):3–4

Bajnok I (1988) Specialization meets entry to practice. *Can Nurs* **84**(6):23–4

Benner P (1984) *From Novice to Expert.* Addison-Wesley, London

Burgoyne S (1992) Emergency nurse practitioners. *Nurs Stand* **6**(27):12

Calkin J (1984) A model for Advanced Nursing Practice *J Nurs Admin* **14** (1):24–30

Casey N (1995) Editorial. *Nurs Stand* **9**(46):3

Castledine G (1994) Specialist and advanced nursing and the scope of practice. In: Hunt G, Wainwright P, eds. *Expanding the role of the nurse:The scope of professional practice,* Blackwell Scientific Publications, Oxford:101-113

Castledine G (1995) Will the nurse practitioner be a mini doctor or a maxi nurse? *Br J Nurs* **4**(16):938–9

Castledine G (1996) The role and criteria of an advanced nurse practitioner. *Br J Nurs* **5**(5):288–9

Chickadonz G, Perry A (1985) Clinical specialization versus generalization: Perspectives for the future. In: McCloskey J, Grace H, eds. *Current Issues in Nursing* 2nd edn, Blackwell Scientific, Boston:73–90

Cooper D, Sparacino P (1990) Acquiring, implementing and evaluating the clinical nurse specialist role. In: Sparacino P, Cooper D, Minarik P eds. *The Clinical Nurse Specialist: Implementation and Impact,* Appleton and Lange, Norwalk, Connecticut: 41–75

Crabtree M (1979) Effective utilization of clinical nurse specialists within the organisational structure of hospital nursing services. *Nurs Admin Quart* **4**:1–10

Davies B, Hughes A (1995) Clarification of advanced nursing practice: Characteristics and competencies. *Clin Nurs Spec* **9**(3):156–60

Dillon A, George S (1997) Advanced neonatal nurse practitioners in the United Kingdom: where are they and what do they do? *J Adv Nurs* **25**:257–64

Ditzenberger G, Collins S, Banta-Wright S (1995) Combining the role of clinical nurse specialist and neonatal nurse practitioner: The experience in one academic tertiary care setting. *J Peri Neo Nurs* **9**(3):45–52

Doherty L (1996) The Advanced Neonatal Nurse Practitioner: Room for one more? *J Neo Nurs* October:23–27

Fenton M, Brykczynski K (1993) Qualitative Distinctions and Similarities in the Practice of Clinical Nurse Specialists and Nurse Practitioners *J Prof Nurs* **9**(6):313–26

Ford L (1979) A nurse for all settings: The nurse practitioner. *Nurs Outlook* **27**(8):516–21

Ford L, Silver H (1967) Expanded role of the nurse in child care. *Nurs Outlook* **15**:43–5

Garland T, Marchione J (1982) A framework for analysing the role of the nurse practitioner. *Adv in Nurs Science* **4**(2):19–29

Gibbon B, Luker K (1995) Uncharted territory: Masters preparation as a foundation for nurse clinicians. *Nurs Ed Today* **15**:164–9

Goodman I (1998) Evaluation and evolution: the contribution of the advanced nurse practitioner to cancer care. In: Rolfe G, Fulbrook P eds. *Advanced Nursing Practice.* Butterworth Heinemann, Oxford:145–65

Greenhalgh and Company Management Consultants (1994) *The Interface Between Junior Doctors And Nurses.* Greenhalgh and Company Ltd

Hamric A (1989) History and Overview of the CNS Role. In: Hamric A, Spross J eds. *The Clinical Nurse Specialist in Theory and Practice, 2nd ed.* W B Saunders, Philadelphia: 3–18

Hanson C, Martin L (1990) The nurse practitioner and clinical nurse specialist: Should the roles be merged? *J Am Acad Nurs Pract* **2**(1):2–9

Hill J (1992) A nurse practitioner rheumatology clinic. *Nurs Stand* **7** (11):35–7

Holt F (1984) A theoretical model for clinical nurse specialist practice. *Nurs healthcare* **5**:445–9

Howie P (1992) Development of the nurse practitioner. *Nurs Stand* **6** (27):10–11

Hunsberger M, Mitchell A, Blatz S *et al* (1992) Definition of an advanced nursing practice role in the NICU: the clinical nurse specialist/neonatal practitioner. *Clin Nurs Spec* **6**(2):91–5

Jones G (1994) Accident and emergency and the nurse practitioner. In: Hunt G, Wainwright P, eds. *Expanding the role of the nurse: The scope of professional practice,* Blackwell Scientific Publications, Oxford:162–81

Joynes J. (1996) An analysis of component parts of advanced nursing practice in relation to acute renal care in intensive care. *Intens Crit Care Nurs* **12**:113–19

Keane A, Richmond T, Kaiser L (1994) Critical Care Nurse Practitioners: Evolution of the Advanced Practice Nursing Role. *Am J Crit Care* **3** (3):232–7

King K, Parinello K, Baggs J (1996) Collaboration and Advanced Practice Nursing In: Hickey J, Ouimette R, Venegoni S eds. *Advanced practice nursing: changing roles and clinical applications.* Lippencott, Philadelphia:146–62

Kitzman H (1989) The CNS and the nurse practitioner. In: Hamric A, Spross J, eds. *The Clinical Nurse Specialist in Theory and Practice,2nd ed.*W B Saunders, Philadelphia:379–94

Manley K (1993) The Clinical Nurse Specialist *Surg Nurs* **6**(3):21–5

Manley K (1996) Advanced practice is not about medicalising nursing roles *Nurs Crit Care* **1**(2):56–7

Manley K (1997) A conceptual framework for advanced practice: an action research project operationalizing and advanced practitioner / consultant nurse role. *J Clin Nurs* **6**:179–90

Mathieson A (1996) Anger at 'mini-doctor' jibe. *Nurs Standard* **10**(50):15

McLoughlin S (1992) Congress on nursing practice meets. *Am Nurs* **24**:23

Menard S (1987) The clinical nurse specialist: Historical perspectives. In: Menard S ed. *The Clinical Nurse Specialist,* John Wiley and Sons, New York:1–7

Mills C (1996) The consultant nurse: a model for advanced practice. *NursTimes* **92**(33):36–7

Mirr M (1993) Advanced clinical practice: a reconceptualized role. *AACN* **4** (4):599–602

Monicken D (1995) Consultation in Advanced Practice Nursing. In: Snyder M, Mirr M eds. *Advanced Practice Nursing: A Guide to Professional Development,* Springer Publishing Company, New York:183–95

NHS Executive (1999) Health Service Circular 1999/217, NHS Executive, London

National Organization of Nurse Practitioner Faculties (NONPF) (1990) *Advanced Nursing Practice: Nurse Practitioner Guidelines: Final Report* NONPF, USA

O'Rourke M (1989) Generic professional behaviours: Implications for the clinical nurse specialist role. *Clin Nurs Spec* **3**(2):128–32

Page N, Arena D (1994) Rethinking the merger of the clinical nurse specialist and nurse practitioner roles. *Image: J Nurs Schol* **26**(4):315–18

Patterson C, Haddad B (1992) The advanced nurse practitioner: common attributes. *Can J Nurs Admin* **5**(4):18–22

Pearson L (1995) Annual update of how each state stands on legislative issues affecting advanced nursing practice. *Nurs Pract* **20**(1):13–51

Pickersgill F (1995) A natural extension? *Nurs Times* **91**(30):24–27

Pickler R, Reyna B (1996) Advanced practice nursing in the care of the high-risk infant. *J Peri Neo Nurs* **10**(1):46–53

Roberts-Davies M, Nolan M, Read S *et al* (1998) Realizing specialist and advanced nursing practice: a typology of innovative nursing roles. *Acc Emerg Nurs* **6**:36–40

Russell J, Hezel L (1994) Role analysis of the advanced practice nurse using the neuman healthcare systems model as a framework. *Clin Nurs Spec* **8**(4):215–20

Salkever D, Skinner E, Steinwachs D *et al* (1982) Episode-based efficiency comparisons for physicians and nurse practitioners. *Med Care* **20**:143–53

Simon P (1992) Pioneer spirit. *Nurs Times* **88**(30):16–17

Smith M (1995) The core of advanced practice nursing. *Nurs Science Quart* **8**(1):2–3

Smith S (1996) Independent nurse practitioner. *Nurs Clin North Am* **31** (3):549–63

Snyder M, Yen M (1995) Characteristics of the advanced practice nurse. In: Snyder M, Mirr M eds. *Advanced Practice Nursing: A Guide to Professional Development,* Springer Publishing Company, New York:3–12

Sox H (1979) Quality of patient care by nurse practitioners and physicians' assistants: a ten year perspective. *Ann Int Med* **91**:459–68

Sparacino P, Cooper D (1990) The role components. In: Sparacino P, Cooper D, Minarik P eds. *The Clinical Nurse Specialist: Implementation and Impact.* Appleton and Lange, Norwalk, Connecticut: 11–35

Spitzer W, Sacket D, Sibley J *et al* (1974) The Burlington randomised trial of the nurse practitioner. *New Eng J Med* **290**:251–56

Spross J, Baggerley J (1989) Models of advanced nursing practice. In: Hamric A, Spross J eds. *The Clinical Nurse Specialist in Theory and Practice* WB Saunders, Philadelphia: 19–40

Stilwell B, Greenfield S, Drury M *et al* (1987) A nurse practitioner in general practice: working style and pattern of consultations. *J Royal Col Gen Pract* **37**:154–57

Sutton F, Smith C (1995) Advanced nursing practice: new ideas and new perspectives. *J Adv Nurs* **21**(6):1037–43

Thibodeau J, Hawkins J (1994) Moving toward a nursing model in advanced practice. *West J Nurs Res* **16**(2):205–18

Torn A, McNichol E (1998) A qualitative study utilzing a focus group to explore the role and concept of the nurse practitioner. *J Adv Nurs* **27**:1202–11

Touche Ross Management Consultants (1995) *Evaluation of Nurse Practitioner Pilot Projects: Executive Summary.* Touche Ross

Tuthill V (1995) The training of nurse surgical assistants. *Br J Nurs* **4** (21):1240–5

Uckan E, Surratt N, Troiano N (1994) Critical care obstetrics: The role of advanced practice nursing. *J Peri Neo Nurs.* **8**(2):40–7

United Kingdom Central Council for Nursing, Midwifery and Health Visiting (1994a) *The Council's Standards for Education and Practice Following Registration.* Annex 1 to Registrar's letter 20/1994, UKCC, London

United Kingdom Central Council for Nursing, Midwifery and Health Visiting (1994b) *Register No 14, Spring.* UKCC, London

United Kingdom Central Council for Nursing, Midwifery and Health Visiting (1994c) *The Future of Professional Practice - The Council's Standards for Education and Practice Following Registration.* UKCC, London

United Kingdom Central Council for Nursing, Midwifery and Health Visiting (1997a)*Register No 19, Spring.* UKCC, London

United Kingdom Central Council for Nursing, Midwifery and Health Visiting (1997b) *The Council's Decision on PREP and Advanced Practice* Registrar's Letter 8/1997, UKCC, London

United Kingdom Central Council for Nursing, Midwifery and Health Visiting (1998) *A Higher Level Of Practice: Consultation Document.* UKCC, London

United States Congress, Office of Technology Assessment (1986) *Nurse Practitioners, Physician Assistants And Certified Nurse Midwives: A Policy Analysis.* Government Printing Office, Washington D.C.

Watson S (1994) An exploratory study into a methodology for the examination of decision making by nurses in the clinical area. *J Adv Nurs* **20**(2):351–60

Watts R, Hanson M, Burke K *et al* (1996) The critical care nurse practitioner: an advanced practice role for the critical care nurse. *Dim Crit Care Nurs* **15**(1):48–6

Wolf G A (1990) Clinical nurse specialists: The second generation. *J Nurs Admin* **20**(5):236–41

Woods L (1997) Conceptualizing advanced nursing practice: curriculum issues to consider in the educational preparation of advanced practice nurses in the UK. *J Adv Nurs* **25**:820–28

Wright S (1994) The nurse consultant: fact or fiction? In: Humphris D, ed. *The Clinical Nurse Specialist: Issues in practice.* MacMillan Press, London. 84–93

2

Expertise and expert practice

Any discussion of advanced nursing practice will, at some stage, inevitably make reference to the concept of clinical expertise and the idea of the expert practitioner. This chapter takes a detailed look at some of the major issues concerning the definition and recognition of expertise and clinical experts in nursing. It examines the criteria commonly used to determine the presence of expertise, as well as exploring some of the more abstract explanations of how experts think and arrive at making decisions.

The trend for discussing the notion of expert practitioners in a nursing context has gained popularity since the mid 1980's and has now become commonplace (Jasper, 1994). While these concepts have generated considerable debate and controversy in the nursing literature in recent years, the long-standing dilemma of how best to explain expert behaviour remains (Rolfe, 1997). While the term expert generally refers to a limited number of individuals who possess certain traits and abilities, it has been suggested that clinical expertise is an essential attribute of nurses at all levels in the organisation (Radke *et al,* 1990). In this context, expertise is not intended to convey the idea that all nurses are necessarily perceived of as experts, but that the development of knowledge and skills to enable practitioners to become more clinically competent is desirable. This serves to illustrate that while the terms expert and expertise are commonly employed in nursing (Jasper, 1994), their usage can generate confusion.

Defining the concept of expertise

A simple dictionary definition states that expertise means:

> ' "...*special skill, knowledge or judgement; expertness", while an expert is a "person who has extensive skill or knowledge in a particular field".*' (Collins English Dictionary, 1986)

A further definition identifies that the relevant skills and/or knowledge are gained via experience (Oxford English Dictionary; 1961). These relatively straightforward definitions yield four attributes of expertise. To be considered an expert, an individual is expected to be:

- skilled
- knowledgeable
- experienced
- identified with a particular field or subject.

When examining the nursing literature on the subject of expertise, there is a consensus that each of these attributes is used to identify the expert practitioner (Benner, 1984; Thompson *et al*, 1990; Benner *et al*, 1992; Jarvis, 1992a). However, in order for expertise to be acknowledged, the four attributes outlined above appear to rely heavily on subjective interpretation to help distinguish the characteristics of experts from non-expert practitioners. It has been suggested that this process relies on some kind of externally validated criterion (Jasper, 1994) to judge the presence of expertise. On reviewing the literature and after conducting a study with a small number of nurses, Jasper (1994) concluded that the defining attributes of the expert were:

- possession of a specialised body of knowledge or skill
- extensive experience in the field of practice
- acknowledgement by others
- highly developed levels of pattern recognition.

This list provides additional attributes to those extracted from the simple dictionary definitions at the outset. While the first two can be seen to support the commonly held characteristics of expertise identified in numerous definitions, the third relates to the notion of recognition and acknowledgement of expertise, while the fourth is more concerned with the cognitive processes in which experts engage. This list of attributes serves as a useful conceptual framework upon which to examine the literature in an attempt to elicit the essential nature of expertise in nursing.

Specialised body of knowledge for expertise

The majority of definitions recognise that an essential characteristic of the expert practitioner is a substantial knowledge base in a particular sphere of practice. In nursing, experts are seen to draw on a wide and varied body of knowledge in the delivery of their care (Robinson and Vaughan, 1992). There is a desire for the knowledge base of experts in nursing be made explicit, yet it often appears to be indefinable (Jasper, 1994). Whether the basis of such a body of knowledge is, as suggested, acquired via the formal academic preparation at the undergraduate or post-graduate level (Fenton, 1992), or is accrued over time by exposure to clinical events and situations (Benner, 1984), or is a combination of both, remains equivocal.

It has been argued that the possession of academic qualifications is insufficient in itself to afford someone the designation of expert (Jasper, 1994). Indeed, Benner (1984) argues that knowledge is built up over years of experience in a particular clinical field and implies that formal academic qualifications are not necessarily a pre-requisite to becoming an expert. In this instance, the expert's specialised body of knowledge is believed to be primarily embedded in practice (Benner, 1984). Yet, when exploring the concept of the expert in relation to advanced practice positions, the current accepted belief, both in the UK and abroad, is that a necessary pre-requisite is academic preparation at the master's degree level (Fenton, 1992, UKCC, 1994). This suggests that in the eyes of professional bodies at the very least, an expert's (ie. advanced practitioner) specialised body of knowledge should be underpinned by theoretical knowledge. Definitions of expertise however, emphasise the **possession** of knowledge and/or skill which is not available to non-experts (Jasper, 1994), not the route by which the knowledge is acquired. This begs the question: does it make a difference if expertise is embedded in practice rather than theory?

One potential answer to this question is provided by Calkin's (1984) work. In her model for advanced practice she explains that a disparity exists between the expertise of what she terms *'experts-by-experience'* and nurses who have undergone formal advanced practitioner academic programmes. The main focus of her model concerns the scope of their respective knowledge bases and analytical abilities. While acknowledging that experts-by-experience possess both a comprehensive knowledge base and analytical skills, Calkin (1984) does not believe that these attributes are developed to the same extent as those of advanced nurse practitioners who have undergone formal academic preparation. She concludes that one of the main differences between the two groups is that advanced practitioners use deliberate reasoning processes to draw on their substantial theoretical knowledge base which, in turn, informs their practice. Calkin's (1984) model does however, assume that the advanced practitioner has considerable clinical experience as well as an appropriate academic qualification. As such, she sees a complementarity between experience and academic qualifications in the development of expertise in nursing practice. On the basis of Calkin's (1984) model, one can conclude there are degrees of expertise in clinical practice influenced by the possession of a specialised body of knowledge, the analytical ability of the practitioner, and the nature of the individual's clinical experiences.

Clearly, all nurses, including advanced nurse practitioners, draw on both practical and theoretical knowledge to enable them to practice (Brykczynski, 1989). Furthermore, experience is considered to be especially important in the development of clinical expertise (Schon, 1983; Benner, 1984), in that it has been argued that all learning, even theoretical abstractions, stem from experience (Jarvis, 1995). This premise is based on the belief that the analysis of professional practice helps to generate knowledge not available by textbook approaches (McCaugherty, 1991), through a process of reflective practice (Schon, 1983).

The expert's specialised body of knowledge, therefore, seems to draw upon three inter-related domains of cognition, identified as propositional knowledge, practical knowledge and experiential knowledge (Heron, 1981). The latter two domains are sometimes combined and referred to as 'tacit' knowledge (Polanyi, 1966). Logic would imply that it is the extent to which each of these domains is developed his/her defines an expert's specialised body of knowledge and thus their expertise. Unfortunately, there is little consensus to be found in the literature regarding what constitutes expert knowledge and the process through which it is acquired.

Propositional knowledge deals with theories, facts and concepts, and has been described as 'textbook' knowledge (Burnard, 1987). In the literature, this is more commonly referred to as Ryle's (1949) concept of 'knowing that'. In Calkin's (1984) discussion of the practice of experts-by-experience, it is this domain of knowledge that she perceives is least well-developed and which she claims is responsible in part for the inability of some experts to be able to account for their actions.

Practical knowledge, or the concept of 'knowing how' (Ryle, 1949), is associated with the acquisition and development of skills and:

'...is the substance of a smooth performance of a practical or interpersonal skill.' (Burnard, 1987, p190)

One could legitimately argue that practical knowledge could be developed in the absence of propositional knowledge, for example, by rote learning of a particular skill. By deduction, one might conclude that practical knowledge in and of itself is a poor indicator of the presence of clinical expertise. This conclusion appears to be supported by the literature, as most writers veer away from describing expertise or experts solely in terms of a set of technical competencies or unique skills, although the possession of specialised skills is acknowledged (Jasper, 1994).

Finally, experiential knowledge is said to be:

'...knowledge gained through direct personal encounter with a subject, person or a thing. It is the subjective and affective

nature of that encounter that contributes to this sort of knowledge.' (Burnard, 1987, pp190–1)

Burnard's (1987) definition explains why experiential knowledge, which he suggests is personal and idiosyncratic, is developed and utilised differently by individual nurses. It also lends weight to the prior notion of degrees of expertise. In some quarters, it is asserted that this kind of knowledge is most influential in the practice of experts. Benner (1984), for example, posits that it is the repeated exposure to clinical situations and events (ie. experiential knowledge) that enables expert nurses to practice differently from novice nurses. Yet this personal knowledge, often gained via reflective practice (Schon, 1983), rests firmly at the bottom of the traditional hierarchy of what constitutes professional knowledge (Johns, 1995). Thus, while becoming a valued source of knowledge upon which practitioners base their decisions for taking action in the practice situation (Carr, 1989), there appears to be a tension between the drive to have advanced nurse practitioner programmes at the Master's degree level (UKCC, 1994), where emphasis on propositional knowledge dominates, and the valuing of the tacit knowledge domain.

Cutcliffe (1997) appears to suggest that the inter-relationship between knowledge domains is responsible for the way experts:

'... question, ...critique, and ... do not accept all things at face value, but examine, seek to understand and discover meaning in both theoretical knowledge and experiential practice-based knowledge. They value both sources of knowledge as vital, especially if the two are viewed together.' (Cutcliffe, 1997, p329)

This might lead one to the conclusion that each domain of knowledge should be developed concurrently so as to add to the overall specialised body of knowledge and correspondingly increase the development of expertise. However, this argument presupposes that all sources of knowledge are equally valued. This is clearly not the case. Benner's (1984) interpretation of expertise would suggest that the different knowledge domains do not necessarily need to develop to the same extent. This point of view overlooks an important issue that appears infrequently in the literature concerning expertise, namely, the currency of knowledge and the concept of evidence- based practice. If expertise is embedded in experiential and practical knowledge (Benner, 1984) to the detriment of propositional knowledge, it can be argued the goal of evidence-based practice in nursing may not be achieved. Jarvis (1992b) suggests that practice based on practical knowledge is accepted by practitioners because it is known to work. He concludes that the nature of practical knowledge is, therefore, essentially conservative, as practitioners *'loathe to change it'* because of its perceived effectiveness. Applying this argument to expertise implies that the specialised body of knowledge of the expert risks becoming stagnant and unresponsive to changing needs (ie. conservative) if the propositional knowledge domain is de-valued or ignored.

There is a more fundamental problem that appears to have dogged attempts to uncover the nature of expertise, namely, the problematic nature of measuring such a complex phenomenon. Benner (1984) was one of the first to recognise this problem when she held that expertise was contextual. Her research focused on expert knowledge embedded in practice, rather than upon the expert clinician. It would appear that an expert's specialised body of knowledge is not judged by any objective measure, which would be difficult to define, but by the use of normative referencing by practitioners in the same sphere of practice. In other words, actors in the social setting construct the notion of expertise locally rather than through the use of any agreed criteria. This approach to identifying the presence of expertise can be found in numerous studies (Benner, 1984; Benner *et al*, 1992; Orme and Maggs, 1993; Kitson *et al*, 1993; Guyton-Simmons and Ehrmin, 1994; Butterworth and Bishop, 1995; Greenwood and King, 1995; Cutcliffe, 1997). Therefore, while a specialised body of knowledge is recognised as an essential attribute of the expert, there are fundamental disagreements about what constitutes specialised knowledge, as well as difficulties in measuring and defining the phenomenon. Consequently, additional criteria have been utilised to identify the presence of expertise.

Extensive experience in the field of practice

The second characteristic associated with expertise is considered to be extensive experience in the field of practice. This attribute identifies three separate features: longevity of service; the scope and range of experiences encountered; and specialisation in a particular field of practice. Taking the first two concepts, it would appear that it is not necessarily longevity of service that promotes expertise, but the nature of the experience that is key (Benner, 1984; Kahneman and Tversky, 1990). In other words, it is how the experience contributes to the development of the different knowledge domains (especially the experiential domain) which appears to be important, and not necessarily how long one has practised in a particular clinical setting. However, many studies, which have relied on the selection of expert participants as part of their methodology, choose duration of experience as one of their prime inclusion criteria. Most commonly, a minimum period of 5 years clinical experience is specified as being desirable, although this figure appears to have been arrived at completely arbitrarily (Benner, 1984; Benner *et al*, 1992; Orme and Maggs, 1993; Butterworth and Bishop, 1995; Cutcliffe, 1997). There is, however, no real consensus on this point and other writers either extend the period of experience required, eg. 8 years (Castledine, 1996) or reduce it accordingly, eg. 18 months (Corcoran, 1986). Still others appear to recognise the uncertain and individual nature of experience by suggesting that a range of durations should be considered, eg. 4–8 years experience (Greenwood and King, 1995).

The positive correlation between length of experience and the development of expertise has an appealing logic. While evidence suggests that expertise does in fact increase over time, there are additional requirements which need to be met (Fox-Young, 1995). The foundation of this argument can be found in Jasper's (1994) assertion that there is no ' *...certain measure of what ... experience consists of, and what experience counts as valid'* (p772).

One has to conclude that it is the individual's personal characteristics and the nature of their experience, rather than the duration of that experience, which is of importance.

The second feature of this attribute concerns the assertion that experience needs to be gained in a 'specific field' of practice. What is unclear however, is how a specific field is defined. For example, does specific relate solely to a narrow field of specialisation, such as coronary care nursing, neonatal nursing, or oncology nursing, where the parameters to the specialised body of knowledge are well defined, or can it relate to more generalist practitioners? In the USA, advanced practitioners include nurse practitioners who work in primary care and whose body of knowledge, by the nature of their client group, is required to be much broader than that of their colleagues working in acute specialisms. Likewise, in the UK, there are master's degree programmes aimed to prepare advanced practitioners to take on a more generic role in both primary and secondary care settings (Gibbon and Luker, 1995). These nurses are perceived to be advanced practitioners and by implication, experts in their fields, yet their knowledge base may not be developed to the same depth as expert practitioners in other specialisms. Arguably, in such cases, the generalist's strength is in his/her breadth of knowledge. Benner and Tanner's (1987) assertion that experts can only function at their highest level within their own speciality, whatever that maybe, appears a sensible way of reconciling the apparent disparity between 'depth' and 'breadth' of knowledge. The premise being that an expert's knowledge base is not transferable to another speciality. Therefore, while experience and the nature of experience are widely acknowledged in the literature as being important factors in determining expertise, it has been suggested that additional criteria need to be made explicit for expertise to be recognised (English, 1993).

Acknowledgement by others

'Many nurses may possess a specialist knowledge base, or have practised a long time in a particular speciality, but not all nurses possessing these two features will be regarded as expert.' (Jasper, 1994, p772)

This brief quotation raises the third criterion of expert practice, namely, the acknowledgement of expertise by others. This issue raises two questions in particular; who identifies the expert? And, are explicit criteria used to inform such a judgement? There appear to be conflicting views in the literature as to whom is best placed to judge if a nurse has acquired expert status and, if adequate criteria exist to help those making the judgement to arrive at such a conclusion.

Benner (1984) and Benner *et al*, (1992) selected their expert participants by the use of peer and supervisor nomination. While some supporters of Benner's work find this strategy quite appropriate (Darbyshire, 1994), critics claim that other stakeholders in healthcare, including health service managers (English, 1993) and even the patient community (Paley, 1996) are equally capable of making judgements about the expertise of nurses. Benner and her colleagues make no claims to the contrary and as such, criticisms based on the unverified assumption that they rejected these communities in favour of the professional peer group appear groundless. On reviewing Benner's work (Benner, 1984; Benner *et al*, 1992), it appears that the choice of peers to select the expert subjects was based as much on methodological pragmatism as on any other criteria.

Likewise, in a UK study of practice experts (Butterworth and Bishop, 1995), nurse executives were given the task of identifying expert practitioners. The criteria they were given to help them identify appropriate nurses and midwives were; length of clinical experience (greater than 5 years), a grade of 'F' or above in the grading structure, and lastly, the subjective judgement of the nurse advisor to nominate someone they believed to be a 'skilled clinician' and expert. While the authors acknowledge that the selection process was open to bias and limitation, especially with regard to the last criterion, the absence of any other suitable criteria in defining expertise becomes evident. Likewise, in an Australian study (Greenwood and King, 1995) the criteria utilised for identifying experts were similar and equally subjective. The feature these strategies have in common are attempts at objective measurements about the person, ie. the number of years experience in a particular field, specific qualifications, a specific grade, and so on, but subjective criteria about their practice expertise and knowledge base.

Perhaps for the moment the question should change from 'What criteria are used to identify the expert?' To ' Who should identify the expert?' Jasper (1994) asserts that the label of expert should be assigned from within the nursing profession, as she believes that: '...only similarly qualified nurses...will be able to identify the true expert' (p773), as they are more likely to understand the role (Fox-Young, 1995). This principle has been followed in a number of international studies which have required expert participants to be identified as part of their methodology (Benner, 1984; Benner *et al*, 1992 Kitson *et al*, 1993; Guyton-Simmons and Ehrmin, 1994: Butterworth and Bishop, 1995; Greenwood and King, 1995; Conway, 1996). Jasper (1994) also acknowledges the importance of recognition from outside the nursing profession for those nurses identified as experts by their peers. Legitimising who outside the nursing profession is best placed to make judgements about the expertise of nurses is, however, not without its problems. This point is illustrated by Cash (1995) in a critique of Benner's (1984) work, when being critical of the use of a non-nurse investigators in the research team assigned to code data relating to expert nursing practice. Cash (1995) concluded that,

> '...the determination of what constitutes expert practice is by the approval of a specific group that is empowered to do so, either by being the research team, managers, or some other legitimising groups. The concept of expertise is therefore arbitrary; it is legitimated by groups or individuals whose status is defined socially.' (p532)

It is the characteristic of expertise being socially constructed by some elite, or invisible process, that has led to the desire for criteria to be developed whereby expertise can be measured and viewed objectively. English (1993) argues that an accurate description of expertise and of the criteria defining excellence are required if nurses are to strive for excellence and presumably identify when it has been achieved. This latter point appears to have merit, as in Bishop and

Butterworth's (1995) study of expert nurses, one respondent is quoted as stating *'I'm surprised that I've been nominated as an expert, no one has bothered to tell me before'* (p30).

The difficulties inherent in such an undertaking are made explicit by Fox-Young (1995) who dedicates an entire paper to outlining the multifarious factors which would require consideration. She recognises that even if appropriate standards and methods could be devised to accurately measure expertise, the interpretation of such data is fraught with difficulty. Elsewhere, it has been acknowledged that it is the tacit domain of knowledge that is at the heart of these methodological problems (Meerabeau, 1992). Consequently, while appearing to call for expert practice to be objectively measured, Fox-Young's (1995) position seems to support Darbyshire's (1994) conclusion that attempts at objective measurement are likely to end in failure as the complex nature and dynamics of the phenomenon do not lend themselves to *'...formal representational propositions which will predict or identify the 'criteria' of expertise'* (Darbyshire, 1994, p757).

In the absence of any agreed or objective criteria, the most visible criterion by which one is judged an expert,

> *'...appear to be the practical abilities which are grounded in a knowledge base. As all other criteria derive from these, it is not only important to possess these capabilities, but it is vital that these are witnessed and labelled as expert by others.'*
> (Jasper, 1994, p773)

Thus, the expert nurse is one who is seen to have the *'capacity to contextualize and to 'adjust' what she knows to particular cases'* (Paul and Heaslip, 1995, p40). The visible criteria may include such things as the expert being seen to be able to perform their craft at a higher standard than most others and to be both effective and efficient (Thompson, *et al*, 1990). In other words, acknowledgement of expertise appears to be by the process of normative referencing, as opposed to criterion referencing. That is, expertise is only constructed in the social setting when it is compared with the meaning of novice in the same setting (Edwards, 1998). As Conway (1996) points out *'much as beauty is in the eye of the beholder, so too is expertise'*. The nature of normative referencing by one's colleagues in a particular setting has the effect of contextualizing expertise, which is the point that Benner (1984) and her colleagues attempt to make explicit and for which they have been derided (Cash, 1995).

While the criterion for judging expertise may be vague at best, the significance of other professional groups identifying expert practice of nurses appears to do with the validation of nursing as a 'major' profession (Jasper, 1994). Arguably, the UKCC's (1994) original expectation for advanced practitioners to be academically prepared at the master's degree level can be seen to serve two purposes. Firstly, to provide practitioners with sound theoretical principles upon which to base their practice, but secondly, to increase the likelihood of advanced practitioners being formally recognised professionally for their clinical expertise and knowledge base.

Highly developed levels of pattern recognition and intuition

While the criteria utilised to identify clinical expertise and experts are only partially made explicit in the literature, it is the cognitive processes which differentiate expert practice from non-expert practice, that have generated greatest interest both within and outside nursing for a number of years. While all nurses possess practical and theoretical knowledge, the way such knowledge is put to use differs according to the degree of competency and expertise of the individual practitioner. It is this process that is believed to separate the expert nurse from any other.

Pattern recognition is for Jasper (1994) what characterises the cognitive processes of the expert practitioner.

' Crucial to this attribute is the development of 'intuitive' patterns of functioning which allow for rapid decision-making ... The mark of the expert is the capacity to think in 'wholes' due to the sophistication of the internalization of knowledge and skills.' (Jasper, 1994, p772)

In other words, it is the internalization of knowledge and skills, combined with the exposure to similar experiences that influence the intuitive patterns of thinking. This view is in accordance with Dreyfus and Dreyfus's (1986) model of intuitive judgement which, has as two of its components, pattern recognition and similarity recognition. While this interpretation bears a strong similarity to Benner's (1984) conclusions, the cognitive processes that underpin and enable the expert to function in such a way remain obscure.

Attempts to explain the concept of expertise, by those perceived as experts, has often proven difficult. Expert nurses commonly articulate that their clinical judgements and decision making are informed by 'gut feelings', 'a sense of uneasiness', or simply by 'vague hunches' (Benner, 1984; Farrington, 1993). It is their inarticulateness that is problematical, but as Schon (1983) states, this is not unusual in that many practitioners make clinical judgements for which they cannot state the criteria or rules that informed their decision. This difficulty in articulating the cognitive processes underpinning clinical decisions has led to criticism. Advances in computer science and the development of so called 'expert systems' modelled on the idea of 'fuzzy logic' provide a further explanation of how expertise is informed by pattern recognition and intuition. Rolfe (1997) explains that in such systems, computers are not programmed with a set of concrete instructions which follow analytic logic. Instead they are programmed with what he calls *'fuzzy rules'* which are much more ambiguous and imprecise. To explain these fuzzy rules he provides the illustration of where a computer might follow an instruction such as, 'a bit to the right' or 'a little higher', as opposed to a precise instruction. He credits a computer scientist called Kosko (1994) with making this breakthrough which has enabled the computer to learn from what experts *do*, rather than relying on experts to verbalise their actions, which often they are unable to do. The benefit of such a development is seen as being that,

> ' *The computer ... has access to the same accumulation of experience, the same thousands of special cases, as ... human experts. Furthermore, it generates its own fuzzy rules based on those experiences **and** is able to verbalise them.* (Rolfe, 1997, p1072, original emphasis)

The actual processes and algorithms the computer uses to mimic expertise are in effect intuitive and based upon weighing up a specific situation and taking a fuzzy weighted average of all the available rules to help determine the appropriate course of action (Rolfe, 1997). Fuzzy logic may help to explain the cognitive processes in which experts engage, in context of the three knowledge domains discussed earlier. For example, the expert nurse combines her theoretical knowledge (propositional knowledge) with her experience of similar situations and cases (experiential knowledge) and her personal knowledge of the situation and its demands (practical knowledge) to 'weigh up' the best course of action she should take. Priority, or the weight assigned to each domain of knowledge, will vary according to individual situations. In a particular situation, an expert may give low priority to the propositional knowledge at her disposal in favour of her experiential and practical knowledge. At other times, the reverse may be true. In this model experts are in effect utilising fuzzy logic as a basis for their practice. The degree of expertise or the accuracy of conclusions and interventions will depend upon the ' *... personal* *knowledge of [the]...individual case, on the volume and diversity of [their]...past experience and on how much scientific knowledge and theory [they]... have at [their]...disposal.'* (Rolfe, 1997, p1074).

By thinking in these terms, Rolfe (1997) suggests that experts should be better placed to articulate the cognitive processes that guide their actions, although it could be argued that the two things do not necessarily go together. It also provides insight into how the cognitive processes of expert nurses differ from those of novice nurses. In effect, this model makes clear the processes to which Benner (1984) alludes in her discussion of intuition and expertise. It also helps to explain the *variance* in degrees of expertise, which is possessed by the individual nurse.

Conclusion

Arriving at a consensus regarding the concept of expertise and its place in nursing is clearly problematic. There is general acknow-ledgement that Benner's (1984) seminal work in this area and its application to a nursing context has promoted considerable debate and has provided a basis upon which to examine the concept more closely. Critics of her work argue that the notion of intuition is so intangible and unscientific that its usefulness in explaining the expertise of nurses is questionable. Moreover, it appears that critics deride Benner's (1984) conclusions because of methodological limitations and her (perceived) failure to fully articulate the cognitive processes that distinguish expert practice from non-expert practice. When Benner's work is viewed within the theoretical frameworks of expert systems (Rolfe, 1997) or cognitive science (Thompson *et al*, 1990) however, she arrives at the same conclusion, only through the use of a different vocabulary and conceptual framework. It can be legitimately argued that she does over-emphasise a reliance on experiential knowledge while playing down the importance of propositional knowledge (Heron, 1981), with one potential complication being that experts may not necessarily base their practice on current knowledge. The fact that experts are not always able to articulate the rationale for their actions and decisions is not necessarily an indicator that one type of knowledge prevails hierarchically or is more refined than another, simply that the cognitive processes involved are difficult to describe. As has been illustrated, it is not the possession of knowledge that designates the expert, but how that knowledge is processed and used to inform clinical practice.

A more contentious issue concerns the formal recognition of expertise and in particular, who should confer the accolade of *expert* on the individual practitioner. It has been argued that expertise needs to be recognised both from within and outside the nursing profession, but the criteria for such recognition cannot be agreed. Benner (1996) acknowledges the power gradient that exists between nursing and medicine and sees the recognition of nursing expertise as being one way to ameliorate the situation. However, one of her critics (Cash, 1995) suggests that until expertise, and intuition in particular, can be located into a positivistic paradigm, such imbalances will remain. As has been illustrated, the difficulties inherent in eliciting objective-based criterion for expertise, other than the crude indicators such as length of service, grade and educational qualifications already in use, appear likely to remain.

Advanced nurse practitioners are frequently referred to in the literature as clinical experts. However, the basis of their expertise is either assumed by virtue of their academic qualifications, or described as a list of competencies that are context bound (Fenton and Brykczynski, 1993). Differentiating the practice of advanced practitioners from that of 'experts-by-experience' is consequently difficult, as experts appear to be classified and recognised by what they *do* and to a lesser extent what they *know*, rather than by a set of definitive characteristics. Calkin (1984) provides one explanation of how the three domains of knowledge are integrated to a greater extent by advanced practitioners than other nurses. What remains unclear from the literature is how nurses move from a position of 'expert by experience' to 'advanced practitioner' and the processes in which they engage whereby they become recognised as an expert. While the importance of propositional knowledge is emphasised in studies of advanced practitioners, the role of intuition as described by Benner (1984) is de-emphasised. There is however an appealing logic that these two concepts are related in some way, which in turn influences how the ANP attends to the needs of the patient in their care. The abstract nature of the concept of intuition remains ambiguous and hence it becomes problematical in terms of understanding its relationships with the other domains of knowledge related to expertise. It is likely that this is one reason why the notion of expertise is socially constructed and recognised. Furthermore, the social learning of expertise that is implicit in the prior discussion cannot be ignored, although there is an absence of literature addressing this subject explicitly.

In attempting to uncover the cognitive process involved in expert action, computer and cognitive scientists have even attempted to explain the phenomenon of expertise from a different perspective (Thompson *et al*, 1990; Rolfe, 1997). However, the actual cognitive processes which differentiate expert practice from that of non-expert practitioners, be it by intuition (Benner, 1984), reflection (Schon, 1983), fuzzy logic (Rolfe, 1997) or organised by a neural network (Thompson *et al*, 1990) remain at best, equivocal. What perhaps becomes more important in understanding the nature of expertise and the expert practitioner is how the individual engages in the transitional process (or social learning) of moving from experienced nurse to advanced (expert) practitioner. It is this fundamental question that will be the focus for the remainder of this book.

References

Benner P (1984) *From Novice to Expert*. Addison-Wesley, London

Benner P (1996) A response by P. Benner to K. Cash, 'Benner and expertise in nursing: a critique'. *Int J Nurs Stud* **33**(6):669–74

Benner P, Tanner C (1987) How expert nurses use intuition. *Am J Nurs* **87**:23–31

Benner P, Tanner C, Chesla C (1992) From beginner to expert: gaining a differentiated clinical world in critical nursing care. *Adv Nurs Science* **14**:13–28

Brykczynski K (1989) An interpretive study describing the clinical judgement of nurse practitioners. *Sch Inq Nurs Pract.* **3**(2):75–104

Burnard P (1987) Towards an epistemological basis for experiential learning in nurse education. *J Adv Nurs* **12**:189–93

Butterworth T, Bishop V (1995) Identifying the characteristics of optimum practice: findings from a survey of practice experts in nursing, midwifery and health visiting. *J Adv Nurs* **22**:24–32

Calkin J (1984) A model for Advanced Nursing Practice *J Nurs Admin* **14**(1):24–30

Carr W (1989) Introduction: understanding quality in teaching. In: Carr W, ed. *Quality in Teaching*. The Falmer Press, Lewes: pp1–20

Cash K (1995) Benner and expertise in nursing: a critique. *Int J Nurs Stud* **32**(6):527–34

Castledine G (1996) The role and criteria of an advanced nurse practitioner. *Br J Nurs* **5**(5):288–9

Collins English Dictionary (1986) Collins, London

Conway J (1996) *Nursing Expertise and Advanced Practice*. Quay Books, Mark Allen Publishing Ltd, Dinton, Wilts

Corcoran S (1986) Task complexity and nursing expertise as factors in decision making. *Nurs Res* **35**:107–12

Cutcliffe J (1997) The nature of expert psychiatric nurse practice: a grounded theory study. *J Clin Nurs* **6**:325–32

Darbyshire P (1994) Skilled expert practice: is it 'all in the mind'? A response to English's critique of Benner's novice to expert model. *J Adv Nurs* **19**:755–61

Dreyfus H, Dreyfus S (1986) *Mind over Machine*. Blackwell Science, Oxford

Edwards B (1998) A and E nurses' constructs on the nature of nursing expertise: a repertory grid technique. *Acc Emerg Nurs* **6**:18–23.

English I (1993) Intuition as a function of the expert nurse: a critique of Benner's novice to expert model. *J Adv Nurs* **18**(3):387–93

Farrington A (1993) Intuition and expert clinical practice in nursing. *Br J Nurs* **2**(4):228–9, 231–3

Fenton M (1992) Education for the advanced practice of clinical nurse specialists. *Onc Nurs Forum* **19**:16–20

Fenton M, Brykczynski K (1993) Qualitative Distinctions and Similarities in the Practice of Clinical Nurse Specialists and Nurse Practitioners *J Prof Nurs* **9**(6):313–26

Fox-Young S (1995) Issues in the assessment of expert nurses: purposes, standards and methods. *Nurs Educ Today* **15**:96–100

Gibbon B, Luker K (1995) Uncharted territory: Masters preparation as a foundation for nurse clinicians. *Nurs Educ Today* **15**:164–9

Greenwood J, King M (1995) Some surprising similarities in the clinical reasoning of 'expert' and 'novice' orthopaedic nurses: report of a study using verbal protocols and protocol analyses. *J Adv Nurs* **22**:907–13

Guyton-Simmons J, Ehrmin J (1994) Problem Solving in Pain Management by Expert Intensive Care Nurses. *Crit Care Nurs* October, 37–44

Heron J (1981) Philosophical basis for a new paradigm. In: Reason P, Rowan J, eds. *Human Inquiry: A Sourcebook of New Paradigm Research.* John Wiley, Chichester

Jarvis P (1992a) Quality in practice: the role of education. *Nurs Educ Today* **12**:3–10

Jarvis P (1992b) Theory and practice and the preparation of teachers of nursing. *Nurs Educ Today.* **12**:258–65

Jarvis P (1995) Towards a philosophical understanding of mentoring. *Nurs Educ Today* **15**:414–19

Jasper M (1994) Expert: a discussion of the implications of the concept as used in nursing. *J Adv Nurs* **20**:769–76

Johns C (1995) The value of reflective practice for nursing. *J Clin Nurs* **4**:23–30

Kahneman D, Tversky A (1990) The simulation heuristic. In: Kahneman D, Slovac P, Tversky A, eds. *Judgement Under Uncertainty: Heuristics and Biases.* Cambridge University Press, New York:201–08

Kitson A, Harvey G, Hyndman S *et al* (1993) A comparison of expert and practitioner-derived criteria for post-operative pain management. *J Adv Nurs* **18**:218–33

Kosko B (1994) *Fuzzy Thinking.* Harper Collins, London

McCaugherty D (1991) The use of a teaching model to promote reflection and the experiential integration of theory and practice in first year student nurses: an action research study. *J Adv Nurs* **16**:534–43

Meerabeau L (1992) Tacit nursing knolwedge: an untapped resource or a methodological headache? *J Adv Nurs* **17**:108–12

Orme L, Maggs C (1993) Decision-making in clinical practice: how do expert nurses, midwives and health visitors make decisions? *Nurs Educ Today* **13**:270–76

Oxford English Dictionary (1961) Oxford University Press, Oxford

Paley J (1996) Intuition and expertise: comments on the Benner debate. *J Adv Nurs* **23**:665–71

Paul R, Heaslip P (1995) Critical thinking and intuitive nursing practice. *J Adv Nurs* **22**:40–7

Polanyi M (1966) *The Tacit Dimension.* Routledge and Kegan Paul, London

Radke K, McArt E, Schmitt M *et al* (1990) Administrative preparation of clinical nurse specialists. *J Prof Nurs* **6**:221–8

Robinson K, Vaughan B. (1992) *Knowledge for nursing practice.* Butterworth Heinemann, Oxford

Rolfe G (1997) Science, abduction and the fuzzy nurse: an exploration of expertise. *J Adv Nurs.* **25**:1070–75

Ryle G (1949) *The Concept of Mind.* Penguin, Harmondsworth

Schon D (1983) *The Reflective Practitioner.* Temple Smith, London

Thompson C, Ryan S, Kitzman H (1990) Expertise: the basis for expert system development. *Adv Nurs Science* **13**:1–10

United Kingdom Central Council for Nursing, Midwifery and Health Visiting. (1994) *The Future of Professional Practice — The Council's Standards for Education and Practice Following Registration.* UKCC, London.

3

Investigating the role transition of advanced nurse practitioners

As the previous discussion has illustrated, the role of the advanced nurse practitioner has been the subject of a great deal of debate and research interest in recent years. The general view to emerge over that time suggests that they have made significant and effective contributions to healthcare delivery in a number of countries. The political and professional initiatives taking place in the UK have led to the situation whereby nurses are increasingly likely to be educated and trained to take on advanced practice roles. While such roles have been mapped out in other countries, from a UK perspective, the concept of advanced practice remains a contemporary issue about which little is known or understood. While the literature provides an insight into the various definitions and models of advanced practice, little systematic inquiry has taken place into the transitional process in which experienced nurses engage when training to become advanced nurse practitioners. The majority of writers who have attempted to describe such transitions have relied on anecdotal evidence and presented rather simplistic accounts of what is, in effect, a complex phenomenon. On the other hand, the limited empirical studies which have been undertaken, have, in the main, focused on the outcome of role transition in terms of **what** advanced practitioners are able to **do** when compared to other nurses or medical practitioners. Consequently, relatively little is known about **how** nurses alter their practice and identity during the process of role transition.

While advanced practice roles have become established in other countries, in the UK there is a great deal of ambiguity concerning the entire concept. The issue of how educational institutions and healthcare organisations construct the notion of advanced practice is likely to have significant implications for how practitioners are not only educated, but also how they implement their roles in clinical practice. In the absence of a common frame of reference and limited evidence from international sources, both universities and trusts will need to reconcile the goals of professional development and ambition with political and organisational expediency. It is from this point of view that while a number of inquiries have acknowledged the social context in which practice takes place, few have explored how advanced nursing practice is influenced or constructed from a social perspective when competing professional and political agendas prevail. In these circumstances, the importance of the social context cannot be overstated. It comes as some surprise therefore, that a number of the studies and papers reviewed in the literature provided only a cursory reference to the influence of the social context upon role transition and the development of advanced practice. Arguably, if inquiries gave greater consideration to the social context, they could be of substantial benefit in helping to provide the answers to questions such as, why do particular roles develop in the ways they do? What are the prime factors that influence this process? Do all advanced practitioners learn the same skills, behaviours and roles, or do they vary from institution to institution? Are advanced practitioners adequately prepared both educationally and clinically, for the job they are expected to perform? While there are many questions that remain unanswered with regard to the whole concept of advanced practice in the UK, a number of these issues and problems were addressed in a study conducted between 1996 and 1998 (Woods, 1998).

This chapter describes the research design and methods adopted for the study. It commences with a presentation of the aims of the investigation, followed by a brief outline of the philosophical, epistemological and pragmatic considerations that guided strategic and methodological choices. This is followed by a detailed account of the research strategy, in which the different phases of the study are highlighted and a description of the data collection methods is provided. The chapter concludes by describing the approach used for data management and analysis.

Aims of the study

The general goal of the study was to investigate the experiences of a group of nurses undergoing training to prepare them for the role of advanced nurse practitioners. The study initially had five broad aims:

1. To explore if the educational and clinical preparation of advanced nurse practitioners were considered appropriate and relevant, in terms of both content and academic level, to the role anticipated to be implemented in practice.

2. To gain an understanding of the expectations of advanced practice held by ANPs and their colleagues.

3. To examine the personal and practice development of ANPs during role transition and identify the ways in which their practice and roles differed from that of their nursing colleagues.

4. To identify the ways in which the ANPs' role influenced the practice of professional colleagues in terms of the organisation and delivery of care and, to explore if the ANP was perceived to be practising from a nursing or medical paradigm perspective.

5. To gain an understanding of the factors that facilitated and/or impeded role development and performance and how such variables exerted influence over the transitional process.

The first two aims were the predominant focus for the initial phase of the study, while the latter aims became increasingly relevant as the inquiry progressed. The aims of the study were intentionally defined in broad terms in keeping with the methodological approach adopted (see below). This strategy allowed flexibility in the research design to pursue the central themes and issues as they emerged.

Methodological considerations

The education, training and implementation of advanced nurse practitioners into clinical practice are relatively unique events for the nursing profession in the UK. As with other contemporary events in nursing, it has been suggested that in order to investigate such a phenomenon:

> '...it is essential that any research approach taken to investigate it should do so within its real life context and make full use of data generated from the dynamic nature of the event. It is consequently important that the research approach allows for the use of multiple sources of information so that evidence can be converged to provide a fair and accurate account of the event.' (Ramprogus, 1995, pp65–6)

In so doing, consideration must be given to the participants' experience and interpretation of the situation, which can then be used as a basis for understanding the phenomenon from various perspectives (Ramprogus, 1995).

In light of these methodological considerations a qualitative approach, based within a constructivist paradigm (Lincoln and Guba, 1985; Guba and Lincoln, 1994), was adopted. Broadly speaking, constructivism shares with other interpretive approaches to human inquiry the goal of:

> '...understanding the complex world of the lived experience from the point of view of those who live it. ... The world of lived

reality and situation-specific meanings that constitute the general object of investigation is thought to be constructed by social actors.' (Schwandt, 1994, p118)

Consequently, Lincoln and Guba (1985) assert that realities have to be considered as wholes and cannot be divorced and understood in isolation from their contexts. It is the premise of this book that the concept of 'advanced practice' is socially constructed by actors in the social setting. As such, there are likely to be as many realities of what constitutes advanced practice as there are actors in the social environment, especially given the absence of an agreed definition of the concept in the UK literature. Consequently, the results of any inquiry which sets out to explore such a phenomenon are likely to be strengthened if account is taken of the multiple realities which exist and if the concept is explored from different contexts and perspectives. It is acknowledged, that while not all interpretations of advanced nursing practice will necessarily have equal merit, or provide convergence, it is nonetheless important to explore the construct in its social context and from a relativistic perspective.

Given these methodological considerations and the aims of the inquiry, a collective case study design (Stake, 1995) was adopted as the most appropriate research strategy. Given the aims of the inquiry, these case studies can be categorised as being both descriptive and exploratory in nature (Yin, 1989).

Case studies have acquired various definitions and usages in the literature (Woods, 1997). A case study has been described as:

'...an exploration of a 'bounded system' or a case (or multiple cases) over time through detailed, in depth data collection involving multiple sources of information rich in context.'
(Creswell, 1998, p61)

Woods and Catanzaro (1988), convey the depth of inquiry involved in case study research when they define it as an:

'...intensive, systematic investigation of a single individual, group, community, or some other unit, typically conducted under naturalistic conditions, in which the investigator examines in-depth data related to background, current status, environmental characteristics and interactions.' (p553)

The selection of a collective case study strategy in favour of other approaches, such as a phenomenological or ethnographic study, was based on the characteristics and features of the case study design, given the aims of the inquiry, the phenomenon being investigated and the constructivist paradigm within which it was framed. As a research strategy, the case study focuses on understanding the dynamics present in the social setting (Eisenhardt, 1989). Consequently, case studies are typified by four elements: context, boundaries, time and intensity (Mariano, 1993).

Given the purpose of the investigation, a decision to pursue a multiple, or what Stake (1995) terms a 'collective' case study design (as opposed to a 'single' case design) involving five cases, was taken. While it has been recognised there is no ideal number of cases, it has been suggested that a number between 4 and 10 works well (Eisenhardt, 1989). While the choice in determining the number of case studies to undertake was in part influenced by resource and pragmatic considerations associated with the investigation, it was principally guided by the theoretical replication logic for undertaking multiple case studies, discussed by Yin (1989). In this study, it was predicted that the development and implementation of advanced nursing practice would vary in different organisations and within different clinical specialisms. The design, therefore, utilised the principle of a 'most-different-systems' approach for conducting comparative case studies (Schultz and Kerr, 1986). Thus, in multiple-case study designs, the convergence of evidence is enhanced by asking about the same phenomenon across cases (Gilgun, 1994). That is to say, variation and differences in cases, add depth and increase our understanding of the phenomenon of interest. In so doing, this strategy provides the opportunity for cross-case analysis, as well as within-case analysis that would be denied by the use of a single case study design. Consequently, in this study, not only are the cases multiple in number, but they occur within different clinical specialisms and across different sites. In this sense, each case is used 'instrumentally' to illustrate the central issue of the study (Creswell, 1998), ie. as opposed to a case being selected purely for its intrinsic characteristics (Stake, 1995). The collective case study strategy is, therefore, considered to be appropriate for exploring the same phenomenon, in a diversity of situations, with a number of individuals (Mariano, 1993).

A feature of the case study design is the use of multiple sources of evidence in the data collection and analysis processes (Yin, 1981). However, before data collection commences, careful consideration and explanation needs to be given to defining who or what comprise a 'case'. Deising (1971) noted that the case study design encountered particular problems in delineating the boundaries of the research entity in question. Clearly, the way a case is defined will have a major impact on the conduct and outcome of the research.

Yin (1989) asserts that the definition of a 'case' or 'unit of analysis' should be related to the initial research question. Consequently, in this study, it was decided that each case would comprise not only the advanced practice nurse, who may be perceived of as the 'key' informant, but also the people with whom he or she are considered to be either actively involved, or who have a significant influence upon (or are affected by) either their education and/or practice. *Table 3.1* details the composition of each intended case study.

Table 3.1: The composition of each case
Each case study aimed to comprise: ❖ The Advanced Nurse Practitioner/student — the key informant   ❖ Consultant Preceptor — a work based consultant whose role was anticipated to include supervision and mentorship of the ANP throughout the transitional process   ❖ Directorate Manager (where in post)   ❖ Clinical Nurse Manager   ❖ University Pathway Coordinator – a university lecturer with responsibility for coordinating the practice and learning experieinces specific to the ANPs practice discipline   ❖ A Junior Doctor   ❖ A Nursing Colleague

Sampling strategy

In common with other qualitative research traditions a 'purposeful' or 'theoretical' sampling strategy (Creswell, 1998) was adopted. Purposive sampling is not based upon the principles of probability sampling, where the aim is to obtain a representative sample, but on the selection of cases believed to be rich sources of data (Reed *et al*, 1996). In this way, the goal of theoretical sampling is to choose cases based on their likelihood of replicating or extending emergent theory (Eisenhardt, 1989).

The population for the study comprised a cohort of twenty-five nurses seconded to a one year, full-time Master's degree programme at a UK university. The local National Health Service Executive, who commissioned the programme, gave the university the explicit remit to prepare nurses to take on roles as advanced nurse practitioners. The majority of study population was drawn from five main clinical specialisms:

1. Adult intensive care nursing

2. Accident and emergency nursing

3. Neonatal nursing

4. Gynaecological nursing

5. Rehabilitation nursing.

A significant factor in defining the population for the study, was that at the time only one university within the region ran a Master's degree course specifically designed to prepare nurses based in clinical practice, as advanced nurse practitioners.

A sample of sixteen nurses was willing to be involved in the study. From this sample, five nurses, one from each specialism, were selected to be the focus of longitudinal case studies. Whereas the *number* of cases was determined by estimating what could be realistically achieved within the resources and time frame of the study, the selection of individual cases was based on the principles of the collective case study design and the theoretical sampling strategy described above. Each of the five individuals was selected specifically for their particular interest and relevance to the phenomenon under study (Patton, 1990). The following criteria were utilised to inform the selection process in which the individuals from five different clinical settings were chosen:

- ◆ the clinical speciality in which the nurse worked
- ◆ the part of the region in which they were employed
- ◆ the prior clinical experience of the nurse
- ◆ the educational background of the nurse.

The five individuals who agreed to full access were asked to provide details of the other case study participants (ie. Consultant Preceptor, Directorate Manager, Clinical Nurse Manager, and University Pathway Co-ordinator) who were to be approached.

Research schedule and data collection methods

The strategies used to collect and analyse data within case studies are similar to some of the techniques used in other qualitative designs (Mariano, 1993). Within the tradition of this approach, multiple methods of data collection were adopted for the study (Yin, 1989). These included; interviews, direct observation, and documentary evidence in the form of self-report role development diaries, clinical records, policies and protocols. Each data collection technique was related to specific aims of the study (see *Table 3.2*) and used at different phases of the investigation in order to provide convergence of evidence.

Table 3.2: Relationship between aims of the study and data collection methods	
Aims of the study	**Methods**
1. To explore if the educational and clinical preparation of advanced nurse practitioners were considered appropriate and relevant, in terms of both content and academic level, to the role anticipated to be implemented in practice	Interviews Observation
2. To gain an understanding of the expectations of advanced practice held by ANPs and their colleagues	Interviews
3. To examine the personal and practice development of the ANP during role transition and identify the ways in which their practice and roles differed from that of their nursing colleagues	Observation Diaries Interviews Records
4. To identify the ways in which the advanced nurse practitioner's role influenced the practice of professional colleagues in terms of the organisation and delivery of care and to explore if the ANP was perceived to be practising from a nursing or medical paradigm perspective	Observation Diaries Interviews
5. To gain an understanding of the factors which facilitated and/or impeded role development and performance and how such variables exerted influence over the transitional process	Interviews Observation Diaries

Data collection

Formal data collection began in January 1996, by which time the advanced nurse practitioner students were a third of the way into their educational programme. Delays in gaining access and awaiting ethical approval meant that this was the earliest time that data collection could commence, although initial contact was made with the student cohort shortly after commencement of the Master's programme. Due to the time constraints placed upon the study, its longitudinal nature, and the flexible nature of the case study design (Eisenhardt, 1989), piloting of data collection procedures did not take place, with the exception of the role development diaries (see below). Discussion of the interview schedules and observation strategies did occur with research supervisors and amendments were made following their recommendations. An overview of the research schedule is provided is provided in *Table 3.3*.

Table 3.3: Research schedule		
Phase 1:	Jan-Apr '96	**Interview 1**: With ANP, Consultant Preceptor, Directorate Manager, Clinical Nurse Manager, University Pathway Coordinator
Phase 2:	Jun-Sept '96	**Observation 1**: Clinical practice – during course
Phase 3:	Nov-Apr '97	**Observation 2**: Clinical practice — first 6 months post graduation of the Master's programme
Phase 4:	Oct-Mar '97	**Role Development Diaries** — 6 months post course, case study ANPs plus the remaining ANPs who agreed to participate in the study
Phase 5:	Jan-Mar '97	**Interview 2**: All case participants (see *Table 3.1*)
Phase 6:	Jun-Dec '97	**Observation 3**: Clinical practice — 9 to 15 months post graduation of the Master's programme
Phase 7:	Nov-Jan '98	**Interview 3**: With ANPs, Consultant Preceptors, Nurse Managers
Phase 8:	Jan '98	**Feedback & Verification**: Case summaries sent to individuals for verification and feedback purposes

The adaptive nature of the case study strategy provides the maximum flexibility in data collection, allowing for modification to the research schedule owing to unpredictable changes in circumstances of the case study participants and their environment. As such, case study researchers have the freedom to make adjustments during the data collection process, but as Eisenhardt points out:

'...flexibility is not a licence to be unsystematic. Rather, this flexibility is controlled opportunism in which researchers take

advantage of the uniqueness of a specific case and emergence of new themes to improve resultant theory.' (Eisenhardt, 1989, p539)

In order to maximise the data collected via this design, three principal methods were adopted for this study.

Interviews

Interviews were conducted at three stages of the study (see *Table 3.3*), each involving select case study participants. The aim and focus of the interviews varied with each stage. Initial contact with interview participants was made either via letter or by the ANP on the researcher's behalf. This was followed by a telephone call to confirm that the participant was willing to be interviewed and to arrange a suitable time and venue for the interview to take place. All the participants approached agreed to the initial interview and agreed to follow-up interviews where requested. Interviews took place predominantly at the participants' place of work during their normal working hours. The exceptions to this rule were the ANPs who were interviewed at their homes, place of work, and in two instances, on university premises.

At the first interview, the aims of the study were explained and the participant was given an information sheet for reference. The participant was invited to ask questions about the study and seek additional clarification where necessary. Most questions concerned issues of confidentiality and anonymity and were answered to the participants' satisfaction. The participants then signed a consent form confirming their acceptance to take part in the study and their right to withdraw from the study at any time was confirmed. Consent forms were then signed by the researcher and kept securely with the relevant case study database.

The length of interviews ranged between 35 minutes and 1 hour and 15 minutes, with the mean average being approximately 45 minutes. Each interview was tape recorded for accuracy with the participants' permission. While the participants and focus of the interviews varied with each stage, a basic interview format was retained throughout. This involved engaging the participant in discussion about the main issues of interest. To this end interview schedules consisted of a number of general themes which were to be discussed at each phase of the inquiry. To ensure that the issues of central concern were addressed during interviews a number of detailed open-ended questions were included in each schedule, although these primarily served to act as prompts and reminders for the researcher. The interview schedule was, therefore, used primarily to provide the general direction of the discussion, while at the same time allowing for participants to raise issues which had not necessarily been included on the schedule. Any such points that were raised during the interview were incorporated, where appropriate, into future data collection procedures.

Observation of clinical practice

Observation of clinical practice was used as a method of data collection throughout the study period. However, due to problems with access, observation visits only occurred in three of the five cases. The use of published observation schedules and instruments was not adopted for the purpose of this study on the basis that: i) there were very few instruments available that measured the constructs of interest; ii) those instruments that were available were perceived to be of limited utility in the context of this study; and iii) it was the researcher's belief that such instruments would have a detrimental and limiting effect on the collection and analysis of data, as they were perceived to pre-conceptualise the phenomenon to be observed. That is not to say the observation of clinical practice was haphazard or lacked rigour. On the contrary, each stage of observation served a different purpose and became increasingly focused.

Each period of observation consisted of spending a full or partial shift accompanying the ANPs as they undertook their daily activities. while observing clinical practice, data collection was supplemented by having access to nursing and medical records. In this way the researcher was not only able to observe practice directly, but was also able examine pertinent documentation completed by the advanced practitioner. Furthermore, access to local policies, protocols and guidelines, which had direct bearing on the ANPs' practice was provided during observation visits.

Due to the geographical location of the study sites and unpredictable changes associated with shift work, all visits were arranged in advance with the ANPs.

When undertaking observation visits, the identity of the researcher was made explicit to patients, their relatives and members of nursing and medical staff. While the researcher's role was primarily as passive observer, the ANPs and, on occasion their colleagues, were engaged in conversation throughout the visit about the development and implementation of the ANP role. Furthermore, in addition to the observation of practice, ANPs were sometimes accompanied on coffee and meal breaks.

The main focus for the observation visits was guided by both the study's aims and the results of ongoing data analysis. The documented accounts of observation visits comprised narrative descriptions of the ANPs' clinical practice, relevant events that occurred during the visit and the ANPs' interactions with nursing and medical colleagues. Relevant quotations and discussion excerpts were recorded verbatim at the time of their utterance so as to maximise recall. The notes from observation visits were taken contemporaneously in a small notepad and written up in full the same day so as to maximise the accuracy and recall of data collected during the visit. While the use of the notepad caused initial unease and suspicion, especially from the ANPs' nursing and medical colleagues, its continued use became familiar and accepted[1], particularly by the ANPs themselves. It is acknowledged however that initially the use of the notepad is likely to have exacerbated any alteration in behaviour that occurred due to the researcher's presence.

During observation visits, ANPs were shadowed as they undertook their daily activities. During each phase of observation, the collection of data became increasingly focused and refined following analysis of the previously collected empirical data and a review of extant theory in the literature. This guided data collection toward convergence with the information collected by interviews and from analysis of the role development diaries. The observation schedule for each of the three cases over the duration of the study period is detailed in *Table 3.4*.

Table 3.4: Schedule of observation visits over duration of study		
Case study	**No of Visits**	**Total Observation Time**
1: Respiratory Medicine	15	64 hours 35 mins
3: Neonatal Unit	20	96 hours 40 mins
5: A & E	16	53 hours 50 mins
Total	51	215 hours 05 mins

---

1   Throughout the different observation stages the ANPs were questioned about their feelings of the use of the notepad for recording their activities and conversations. All stated that they had soon become familiar and used to it and did not feel threatened or particularly conscious of its continued use.

Role development diaries

In addition to interviews and observation of clinical practice, the 16 ANPs who initially agreed to participate in the study were asked to maintain a self-report role development diary for the first six months they were in clinical practice following graduation from the Master's degree programme. The aims of the diary were to establish how practice activities, and the factors influencing the development and implementation of the advanced practice role, varied across different clinical environments and health authorities. In so doing, the diaries provided additional data and enhanced the convergence of evidence collected by other means.

The diary construction and format, which was devised following analysis of the first series of interviews and observations, incorporated the key activities of advanced practice as they were perceived and anticipated by the case study participants. Each diary contained entries for five consecutive days in clinical practice. The layout of the diary was such that for each day the ANP was asked to enter information into different sections. In the first section, the ANPs were asked to record the activities in which they had been involved. In addition to documenting daily activities, each day the diary was completed the informant was asked to identify: i) their involvement in any activities or skills which they considered to be either 'new' or 'advanced'; ii) the factors that had helped or hindered them in their practice that day; and iii) provide general comments or an account of a 'critical incident' that for them typified their development or involvement as an advanced practitioner.

Prior to being distributed the diary was piloted with two ANPs in different clinical settings. Each was asked to complete the diary for one week along with a questionnaire pertaining to: the diary layout; the time taken to enter the information being elicited; and the potential usefulness of the diary in auditing ANP practice. Based on the results of piloting, minor modifications were made to the layout of the diary and relevant information integrated into the instructions.

The diaries were sent out to all sixteen ANPs who had originally agreed to participate in the study. The first diaries were distributed for use in October 1996 and the last in March 1997. At the end of each month, a new diary was sent to the ANPs, along with a stamped addressed envelope to encourage return of the previous month's diary. Eleven ANPs, including 3 case study ANPs, complied with the request to maintain a diary.

Summary of data collection strategy

Data was collected from multiple and varied sources. While the data was predominantly qualitative in orientation, some quantitative data was gathered, especially via the role development diaries. This is perfectly consistent with the case study strategy as described by Yin (1989) in that the two types of data can be utilised legitimately in the same study (Cresswell, 1998). In common with other qualitative approaches, case study research shares the characteristic that data collection and data analysis occur simultaneously throughout the duration of the study (Mariano, 1993; Gilgun, 1994; Miles and Huberman, 1994). The use of this strategy helped to inform and direct the focus of future data collection and analysis. In conclusion, the data set for this study was collected via the three main sources, outlined in *Table 3.5*.

Table 3.5: Main data sources		
Method	**Number/duration**	**Source**
Interviews	57/--	Case study participants
Observation	51/215 hrs 05 mins	Case study ANPs
Diaries	52 diaries/246 days	11 ANPs inc. 3 case study ANPs

Data analysis

The analytical strategy adopted for this study was *based* upon the principles of Glaser and Strauss's (1967) grounded theory method, whose procedures and techniques have been further refined by Strauss and Corbin (1990). While various writers suggest their own analytical strategies in the context of the case study design (Lincoln and Guba, 1985; Yin, 1989; Stake, 1995) there is a lack of consensus for the analysis of qualitative data (Creswell, 1998). While the techniques and procedures associated with grounded theory were devised for use specifically within that tradition, they share general characteristics with strategies employed in other qualitative research designs which adopt an inductive approach to data analysis. These techniques include; the generation of codes, the reduction of data, the generation and relating of categories, and the development of analytic frameworks. As such, grounded theory:

> *'...provides a set of analytic techniques that can be seen as representing procedures that are consistent with, or have been assimilated into, most other approaches to qualitative research.'* (McLeod, 1995, p93)

Furthermore, with regard to the research strategy adopted for this study, Annells (1996) points out that it is not uncommon for the grounded theory method to be applied within the constructivist inquiry paradigm. Moreover, others confirm it to be a legitimate analytical strategy that can be used within the case study design (Eisenhardt, 1989; Gilgun, 1994). In this sense, the grounded theory method and techniques utilised in naturalistic inquiry provide a model from which to think and work (Schatzman, 1991) and are not simply procedures or techniques to be adhered to blindly.

It is evident in a study of this size and nature that the sheer volume of data collected can be problematical if management and analysis are not anticipated (Yin, 1989; Woods, 1997). For the purpose of this study, a computer package was utilised to assist in data management and analysis. The software used, QSR NUD-IST (Non-numerical Unstructured Data Indexing Searching and Theorizing), is a powerful index based program which provides extensive coding, retrieval and searching facilities, which aids data storage, management and analysis. Cresswell, (1998) demonstrates how the program, which was designed using grounded theory analysis procedures as a template, can be put to use in five different research traditions, including both grounded theory and case studies. This package was chosen over other programs because of its strength as a powerful indexing and retrieval system and its congruence with the analytical strategy adopted for the inquiry. It is of additional benefit to studies which utilise multiple sources of evidence in data collection (as in this one) and which require a clear and well structured indexing system in order to store and follow the chain of evidence (Yin, 1989). Characteristically, this helps increase the trustworthiness and quality of a case study (Mariano, 1993).

While there are obvious benefits to the use of computer programs in qualitative analysis, a number of disadvantages to their use has also been highlighted. These include: the resource demands on the researcher; the potential for categories to become 'fixed' within the program; and an over reliance on the package to undertake analytical procedures (Cresswell, 1998). While being cognisant of these factors, the details of data analysis procedures adopted in this study are illustrated in the form of an algorithm in *Figure 3.1*.

Figure 3.1: Flow diagram of data management and coding procedures

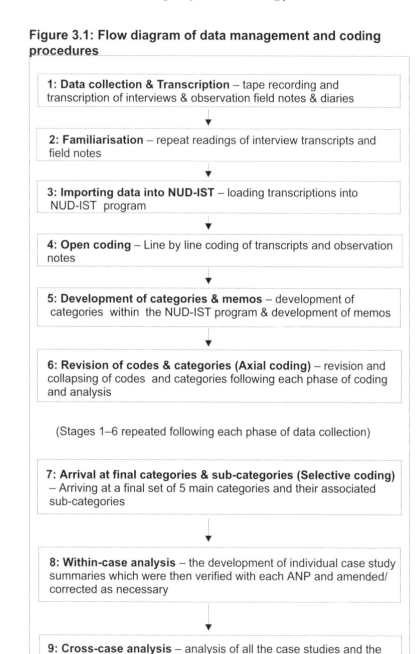

1: Data collection & Transcription – tape recording and transcription of interviews & observation field notes & diaries

2: Familiarisation – repeat readings of interview transcripts and field notes

3: Importing data into NUD-IST – loading transcriptions into NUD-IST program

4: Open coding – Line by line coding of transcripts and observation notes

5: Development of categories & memos – development of categories within the NUD-IST program & development of memos

6: Revision of codes & categories (Axial coding) – revision and collapsing of codes and categories following each phase of coding and analysis

(Stages 1–6 repeated following each phase of data collection)

7: Arrival at final categories & sub-categories (Selective coding) – Arriving at a final set of 5 main categories and their associated sub-categories

8: Within-case analysis – the development of individual case study summaries which were then verified with each ANP and amended/corrected as necessary

9: Cross-case analysis – analysis of all the case studies and the development of cross-case study propositions

Figure 3.1 outlines how data collection and analysis took place throughout the duration of study within a grounded theory framework. Each stage of data collection and analysis is briefly annotated in order to demonstrate how the final set of main categories and associated sub-categories emerged and were developed through a systematic and admittedly time-consuming process. The results of this detailed and extensive analytical procedure are discussed in the subsequent chapters.

References

Annells M (1996) Grounded theory method: philosophical perspectives, paradigm of inquiry, and postmodernism. *Qual Health Res.* **6**(3): 379–93

Creswell J (1998) *Qualitative Inquiry and Research Design: Choosing Among Five Traditions.* Sage Publications, Thousand Oaks, California

Deising P (1971) *Patterns of Discovery in the Social Sciences* Aldine Publishing Company, New York

Eisenhardt K (1989) Building theories from case study research. *Acad Man Review.* **14**(4):532–50

Gilgun J (1994) A Case for case studies in social work research. *Soc Work* **39**(4):371–80

Glaser B, Strauss A (1967) *The Discovery of Grounded Theory* Aldine de Gruyter, New York

Guba E, Lincoln Y (1994) Competing Paradigms in Qualitative Research. In: Denzin N, Lincoln Y eds. *Handbook of Qualitative Research.* Sage Publication, Thousand Oaks, California:105–17

Lincoln Y, Guba E (1985) *Naturalistic Inquiry.* Sage Publications, Newbury Park, California

Mariano C (1993) Case study: the method. *Nat League Nurs* **19**(2535): 311–37

McLeod J (1995) *Doing Counselling Research.* Sage Publications, London

Miles M, Huberman A (1994) *Qualitative Data Analysis, 2nd ed.* Sage Publications, Thousand Oaks, California

Patton M (1990) *Qualitative Evaluation and Research Methods. 2nd ed. Sage* Publications, Newbury Park, California

Ramprogus V (1995) *The Deconstruction of Nursing.* Avebury, Aldershot

Reed J, Proctor S, Murray S (1996) A sampling strategy for qualitative research. *Nurs Res* **3**(4):52–68

Schatzman L (1991) Dimensional analysis: Notes on an alternative approach to the grounding of theory in qualitative research. In: Maines D ed. *Social organization and social process: Essays in honor of Anselm Strauss.* Aldine De Gruyter, New York: 303–14

Schultz P, Kerr (1986) Comparative case study as a strategy for nursing research. In: Chinn P, ed. *Nursing research methodology: Issues and implementation.* Aspen, Rockville, MD: 195–220

Schwandt T (1994) Constructivist, Interpretivist Approaches to Human Inquiry. In: Denzin N, Lincoln Y, eds. *Handbook of Qualitative Research.* Sage Publication, Thousand Oaks, California: 118–37

Stake R (1995) *The Art of Case Study Research.* Sage Publications, Thousand Oaks, California

Strauss A, Corbin J (1990) *Basics of Qualitative Research*: *Grounded Theory Procedures and Techniques.* Sage Publications, Newbury Park

Woods L (1997) Designing and conducting case study research in nursing. *NT Res* **2**(1):48–56

Woods L (1998) *Reconstructing Nursing: A Study of Role Transition in Advanced Nurse Practitioners.* Unpublished PhD Thesis, University of Keele

Woods N, Catanzaro M (1988) *Nursing Research: Theory and Practice.* Mosby, St Louis

Yin R (1981) The case study crisis: some answers. *Admin Science Quart* **26**: 58–65

Yin R (1989) *Case Study Research: Design and Methods (Revised Edition)* Sage Publications, Newbury Park, California

4

Reconstructing nursing

This chapter begins with a brief summary of the central themes to emerge from the findings of the study described in the previous chapter. A detailed explanation of the concept of reconstruction and how it relates to the idea of advanced nursing practice follows. A conceptual model is then presented to illustrate the complex and inter-related nature of the process of role transition. The impact of the social context and how it influences role transition is outlined, revealing the contingent nature and idealised notion of practice reconstruction (Woods, 1999).

Key themes to emerge from the study

The three key themes, which emerged from the findings were:

1. That while the nature of role transition varies in different clinical settings, the process of reconstruction in which practitioners engage can be understood in terms of changes that take place to seven personal and practice domains. The way in which these domains are reconstructed is dependent upon the orientation of role transition.

2. Regardless of clinical setting or practice orientation, the process, rate and parameters of reconstruction are determined by, and contingent upon, locally imposed conditions. The major conditions which affect role transition are: organisational governance; the nature of the clinical environment; the traits and abilities of the individual; the degree of novelty and discretion pertaining to the reconstruction of nursing practice; and the influence of transitional relationships in the practice setting (Woods, 1999).

3. The process of reconstructing a new nursing role results in one of three outcomes [adapted from Nicholson's (1984) theory of work role transition] depending on the nature and influence of the dominant contingent conditions in the practice setting. These operational outcomes have been classified as: practice replication; practice fragmentation; and practice innovation. In addition to the operational outcomes of practice reconstruction, role transition involves the initial stages in the development of a new professional identity whose purpose can be seen to be one of recognition, empowerment and escapism.

These three themes can be seen to have a relationship with one another, which can be illustrated by the use of a conceptual model (*Figure 4.1*). The model indicates an iterative cycle that is intended to demonstrate that the process of reconstruction is dynamic in nature, with changes to any of the variables being possible. So for example, if the nature of contingent conditions changes significantly within the practice environment, there is likely to be equal impact on both the process and outcome of role transition. In this example, changes in contingent conditions could be either favourable or detrimental to the advanced practitioner and hence, her or his practice and the corresponding outcomes would be influenced accordingly.

The problem of definition

Nurses have an established tradition of extending and expanding their practice and skills in a variety of ways. The trend for role expansion clearly indicates an increase in both magnitude and momentum, with a recent Department of Health project mapping out over 800 new roles[1] amongst nurses and professions allied to medicine in acute care settings alone (Cameron, 1998). Moreover, it is becoming increasingly common for nurses who undertake role extension to assume a different job title as an indication that they have undergone additional training, such as in the case of 'emergency nurse practitioners', 'enhanced role nurses' and so on. On closer scrutiny however, it becomes apparent that in many cases nurses have simply incorporated selected additional tasks or skills, often with minimal training, into an already established nursing role. Just one example of this phenomenon is in the case of some early emergency nurse practitioner roles, where nurses were taught to assess and treat minor injuries and in the process learn a limited number of additional skills, such as say suturing and palpation. Role expansion has, of course, occurred along similar lines in a variety of clinical settings, not just in accident and emergency departments. In this type of scenario nurses usually work within strict protocols and guidelines with the level of autonomy and decision making powers being purposely restricted. There are many benefits to these types of role development, not only for nurses, but service organisations and patients.

---

1   New roles in this context were defined by post holders either undertaking activities beyond the accepted scope of practice for a specific professional group, or undertaking completely new work roles.

Figure 4.1: A conceptual model of role reconstruction in advanced nurse practitioners

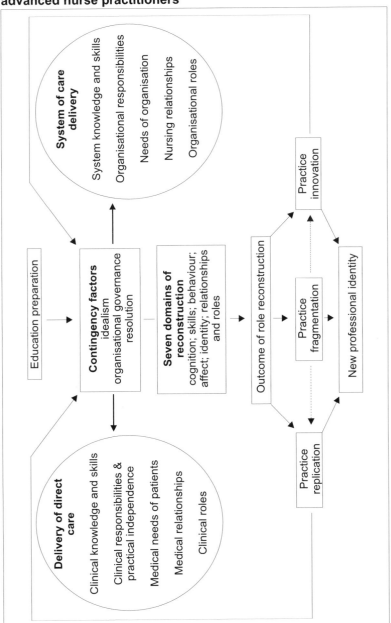

The thorny question is, however, does this type of role development constitute 'advanced' practice? There is no question that such nurses are advancing their practice to the benefit of all concerned, but can their practice be truly called advanced? My response to these types of questions will become apparent in due course.

While identifying a nurse who has developed a limited number of additional skills as an advanced practitioner is at best questionable, is the argument any more compelling in those instances where nurses have taken up new posts involving a radical shift in roles and responsibilities? The relatively new role of the 'surgical assistant' is one such post that can be used to examine this argument. The question one might pose in this example is that while such a practitioner may possess skills clearly absent in nurses in a wider context, do they meet the criteria, whatever they may be, to be classed as an advanced practitioner? The case **against** such a view follows along the lines that the role of the incumbent is no longer involved in the practice of nursing, but acts as a technician who is directly accountable to a medical practitioner. In this instance, the post-holder assumes an identity similar to that of a physician assistant who, as a practitioner, is not necessarily required to have a nursing background. The absence of the term **nurse** from such job titles serves to reinforce the argument that when nurses occupy such positions, which incidentally some consider represent career advancement, the roles in themselves do little to signify any progress or development of the practice of nursing per se. It is easy to see how the problem of definition has pre-occupied professional organisations and individuals in trying to unravel the enigma that is advanced practice.

A different perspective

The educational preparation and implementation of advanced nurse practitioner roles that was the subject of this study represented a major shift in nursing strategy. In this instance, practitioners were required to undertake a Master's degree course whose purpose was to provide them with the foundation and skills from which they were expected to advance nursing practice. Advance in this context was related to the expectation that ANPs would break established nursing boundaries and forge new roles and relationships, rather than simply accept delegated tasks from other disciplines as they have done in the past. An explanation of the concept of reconstruction as a process in which practitioners can be seen to engage during the transition between roles follows.

The process of reconstruction

Studies of role transition in nursing provide little insight or help in understanding the concept of reconstruction as it applies to advanced nurse practitioners in the UK. This is because while transitions have been identified as a central concept in nursing theory (Schumacher and Meleis, 1994), those inquiries that have investigated this phenomenon have done so from a perspective of established roles and stable transitions. For example, the transition from student to staff nurse, where the outcomes and expectations of the process are well known and widely understood, has been the subject of many studies (see: Talarczyk and Millbrandt, 1988; Jairath et al, 1991; Alex and McFarlane, 1992). Likewise, the inquiries that have examined the transition of nurses into advanced practitioner roles, such as clinical nurse specialist and nurse practitioner (Anderson *et al*, 1974; Oda 1977; Lukacs 1982; Hamric and Taylor, 1989; Bass *et al,* 1993; Shea and Selfridge-Thomas, 1997; Brown and Olshansky, 1997; Roberts *et al*, 1997) are predominantly North American in origin and relate to movement between roles which also have been in existence for a number of years. The validity of drawing comparisons between the findings of this study and those cited above is highly questionable, given both the situational differences and novelty of the advanced practice role in the UK. Moreover, the majority of US studies explains the process of transition in terms of a series phases or stages through which role incumbents pass at various points in time. In this sense, the period of transition signifies a 'rite of passage' (Murray, 1998). The idea of practice reconstruction as presented in this text takes somewhat of a different perspective as will become apparent.

In one of the relatively few studies in the UK to explore specialist and advanced nursing practice, Roberts-Davies *et al* (1998) developed a 'typology of innovative nursing roles' from the nursing literature. They developed a number of different 'domains' to identify the characteristics which:

> '...reflect the **main** orientation or emphasis within a given role.' (Roberts-Davies *et al*, 1998, p37 — original emphasis).

This study, along with its American counterparts, appears to have had little concern with the process of **how** nurses reconstruct their practice as advanced practitioners, instead appearing to be pre-occupied with attempting to generate criteria by which specialist and advanced practice can be differentiated. Hence, the taxonomy of domains that was generated was based on: the psychomotor skills performed by the practitioner (ie. the skill/task specific domain); the various roles in which practitioners engaged (ie. role specific domain); the characteristics of the patient population (ie. the condition specific domain); the practice discipline (ie. area specific domain); and other generic areas relating to client groups and the context of care delivery. Likewise, the UKCC appears to have adopted a similar strategy in its generation of a set of pilot standards relating to the notion of a 'higher level of practice' (NHS Executive, 1999). Considerable effort has been put into developing various criteria that will provide practitioners with a set of explicit standards which will need to be met if they are to be recognised as having attained a higher level of practice. The standards fall under an assortment of categories, such as: providing effective healthcare; improving quality and health outcomes; evaluation and research; leading and developing practice; innovation and changing practice and so on. Inevitably, each set of standards is described in terms of a set of behavioural indicators, confirming what a practitioner must be able to **do** within each category. For example, in the category of 'providing effective healthcare', one standard states that practitioners working at a higher level of practice

> *'...assess individuals holistically using a range of different assessment methods and reach valid, reliable and comprehensive patient and client-centred conclusions which manage risk and are appropriate to needs, context and culture.'* (NHS Executive, 1999, 14)

In generating these criteria, albeit only at the pilot stage, the UKCC, to its credit, is attempting to differentiate how the breadth, depth and complexity of a higher level of practice can be differentiated and recognised. While such standards are both desirable and necessary for the profession and as such are welcome, they nonetheless follow the general trend of focusing on what nurses should be able to **do** within certain parameters. On the other hand, the **process** of practice and role development necessary to become recognised as a higher level practitioner, just as with advanced practitioners, remains largely implicit.

It appears from examining the literature then, that previous studies have failed to conceptualise **how** practice is reconstructed when developing a 'new' nursing role. Arguably, this book adopts a relatively unique position in attempting to understand and explain the phenomenon of reconstruction and its relationship to the contingent conditions which determine both the process (ie. the *how*) as well as the outcome (ie. the *what*) of role transition for advanced nurse practitioners.

The ideas of reconstruction and transition are central to this text. Meleis (1986) describes transitions as complex, dynamic processes that occur over time and involve a directional change from one state to another. She goes on to suggest that transitions reflect an internal process of change, whereby alterations in roles, relationships, abilities, identity and behaviour take place. The evidence from my study supports Meleis' conclusions, inasmuch as in the transition from experienced nurse to advanced nurse practitioner, nurses engage in a process of reconstruction involving changes to their practice, their roles, their relationships and their identity. Moreover, practitioners undergo this transformation in the absence of a common frame of reference and without recourse to prior role models. The problems of novelty and ambiguity of practice reconstruction are exacerbated in this instance by the innovation of such roles also being new to the organisations in which the practitioners were employed. Schumacher and Meleis (1994) identify five conditions that influence transitions: the environment; level of planning; knowledge and skill; expectations; and meaning. It is the latter two conditions in particular that give rise to the phenomenon of multiple interpretations and meanings amongst different stakeholders regarding the roles which advanced practitioners are expected to perform and the nature of practice reconstruction (Woods, 1999). This results in a situation whereby the concept of advanced practice is socially constructed by various actors within the organisation, which in turn leads to the phenomenon of an idealised notion of advanced practice. The existence of an idealised notion of advanced practice is one of the main factors that makes the process of reconstruction difficult for advanced practitioners. That is to say, the organisations that desired to see the development of advanced practitioners, as well as ANPs themselves, constructed a set of idealised descriptors of what such a practitioner would be able to accomplish within a given clinical setting. In essence, the outcome of role transition failed, perhaps unsurprisingly, to live up to such an idealised notion (Woods, 1999).

It is the premise of this book that the concept of reconstruction provides a framework which enables the construct of advanced practice to be distinguished from other forms of role development in nursing. During the transition from experienced nurse to advanced practitioner the individual is required to re-build or re-structure the seven domains that comprise and inform nursing practice, which include:

- cognition
- skills

* behaviour
* affect
* identity
* relationships
* roles.

Reconstruction in this sense occurs concurrently along two axes: the **personal** and the **practice**, with each informing and to some extent depending on the other. The latter can be viewed as the outcome (or the *what*) of reconstruction, ie. what is observable and can be seen to have changed in terms of role enactment, while the former involves the process (or the *how*) of reconstruction in which the individual engages on a personal level. In terms of work role transitions these concepts have been referred to elsewhere as 'personal' development and 'role' development (Nicholson, 1984). These two dimensions can be considered discretely or in conjunction with one another. When viewed in relationship with one another, role development should not only be considered to be dependent upon personal development, but also upon the nature of contingent conditions in the clinical setting (Woods, 1999). It is proposed that to understand the concept of reconstruction and advanced practice, one needs to examine fully the context within which role transition takes place. In this sense, the classification of the variables personal and role development serves to be of only theoretical significance. For the purpose of explanation and clarity, each of the seven domains listed above will be discussed discretely, with examplars being provided. In reality however, the developments and changes occurring in each domain should be thought of as being interrelated and interdependent.

Breaking the mould

Integrating new psychomotor skills into practice and having to change an established mind-set, with the concomitant development of cognitive skills and revised ways of thinking, are not inconsiderable feats for nurses to accomplish. The complex nature of advanced practice is such that the idea of merely adding new skills and competencies to an existing professional profile is a gross over-simplification of the reality of changing practice. However, if developing the concept of advanced practice is not just about the addition of new skills and competencies, to what does the process of reconstruction relate? It is the premise of this book that paradoxically, one needs to relate the concept of 'reconstruction' to that of 'deconstruction' to fully appreciate the processes involved in integrating new skills and competencies into a model of advanced practice. This is not immediately evident from the literature. In other words, the process of reconstruction involves the practitioner in initially engaging in an act of 'deconstruction' within each of the seven domains identified above **prior** to their reconstruction at an individual and collective level. This process is necessary in order for the practitioner to accommodate the changes required within each domain, which in turn allow practice to develop at higher level. An everyday analogy may help to clarify this concept.

Consider you are having some building alterations done to your home. Some modifications may be modest and involve minor additions to the existing structure, such as having a new conservatory. In such cases, there are few, if any alterations to the existing structure of the building, except maybe having to move a doorway. This would be analogous to a nurse adding a limited number of additional skills to her repertoire, such as the ability to cannulate. To get back to the building analogy however, some people may have major alterations done to the structure of their home, such as having a two-storey extension. In this scenario builders are required to knock down walls, take out windows, move doors and so on. In other words, parts of the building are *deconstructed*, so that the new extension is able to integrate with the existing structure. The aim of having the building work done is to maximise the utility of your home in new ways that were not possible, prior to the modifications being made. In this sense, the original building has undergone major *reconstruction* combining the new with the old. While some parts of the original building remain intact and untouched, as a domicile it has undergone major transformation. As a result, the new building can be utilised in new and different ways to the original structure, with rooms being used for different purposes, their contents moved, new furniture added and so on.

Getting back to the concepts of advanced practice and reconstruction, it is important to understand that deconstruction is not a destructive process. That is to say that cognition, skills, roles and so on, are not simply jettisoned or rejected during the process of reconstruction. Rather, through the practitioner engaging in deliberate actions and reflection, elements within each domain are selected and modified within the parameters of the new role with the goal of maximising performance. Patient assessment can be used as a general example to illustrate the premise of this argument.

Prior to role transition all the ANPs involved in this study were experienced nurses who were considered to be competent in performing nursing assessments of the patients in their care. Nursing in this context is generally perceived to be primarily concerned with the process of caring (van Maanen, 1990; Graham, 1991; Salussolia, 1997) in which the nurse takes on a series of therapeutic roles which are seen to be largely independent from medicine and the professions allied to medicine. Following role transition however, some of the advanced practitioners in this study found themselves in the position whereby, as part of their new role, they were required to not only undertake nursing assessments of patients, but in addition perform full physical and health assessments. In turn this required that ANPs became competent in the use of new equipment and developed new skills such as inspection, auscultation, percussion and palpation. Changes in their roles and responsibilities demanded they refine not only their psychomotor skills, but also cognitive skills such as clinical judgement and diagnostic interpretation. It was the evaluation of the data collected during the nursing, physical and health assessments of patients that allowed them to arrive at appropriate therapeutic decisions. The following case example will hopefully illustrate this process further.

Prior to developing an advanced practice role, one of the ANPs in the study worked on a gynaecology ward as a deputy ward manager. In her day-to-day activities she conducted numerous nursing assessments of the patients in her care. She routinely took patients' nursing histories, conducted baseline observations and as with many experienced nurses, was able to arrive at a good idea of the nature of patients' problems and their likely treatment and prognosis. However, as part of her role transition in becoming an ANP the same nurse ultimately found herself running an early pregnancy assessment clinic. The clinic, previously conducted by medical staff, aimed to assess and treat women presenting with gynaecological problems during early pregnancy. By the end of the study the ANP was able to integrate a nursing assessment with taking a full medical history and performing a full physical examination of patients who presented. Based on her assessment she would make provisional diagnoses, conduct necessary investigations, arrange for patients to be admitted or discharged and was even able to book the theatre for women requiring surgical interventions. In addition, she was able to spend time with women to provide the necessary counselling and advice that are essential to the nursing care of this group of patients. She did all this autonomously, and only consulted senior physicians when she felt there was a need for a second opinion or advice.

These kinds of changes are not only characteristic of the ANPs in this study, but are evident in the way changes in the practice of advanced practitioners are described in the literature. The process of moving toward a new level of practice competence can be seen to have involved the ANPs in deconstructing their notion of both what constituted patient assessment and what activities should be performed during the intervention. As a process, this was necessary in order to allow the ANPs to accommodate the new concepts and skills, to which they had been exposed, into their practice and cognitive frameworks. Therefore, new skills and activities were not simply performed in isolation to the **nursing** assessment of the patient. Instead, ANPs engaged in a process whereby they reconstructed the concept of patient assessment. They did this by assimilating the new knowledge and competencies they had acquired during their training into their existing cognitive and skill domains, in order to provide a comprehensive and complete assessment of the patient. Thus, reconstruction in this context can be seen to involve the integration of new concepts and skills into an existing framework of understanding. In this sense deconstruction and reconstruction are not processes that occur in strict sequence or instantaneously. Rather, they are gradual in nature, involving the parallel development of specific domains in an iterative cycle as the practitioner is increasingly exposed to more complex role demands.

The evidence from this study supports the notion that ANPs engage in the deconstruction-reconstruction cycle in each of the seven domains identified, according to the orientation of their transition and the specific requirements of the new role. That is to say that different domains are deconstructed and reconstructed at different times, at different rates and by differing degrees according to the demands of role transition and the individual's previous experience. The cycle can be seen to be at its most active at the outset of role transition and decreases in intensity as the incumbent's practice becomes established in their new role. Consequently there is an inverse relationship between reconstruction and deconstruction over the duration of the transition (*Figure 4.2*). This is a concept that has not only emerged from this inquiry, but is one that has been implicit in the findings of other studies. For example, Roberts *et al*, (1997) observed in a sample of nurse practitioner students in the USA that as they progressed in their education and practice they:

'...experienced a re-emergence of their nursing knowledge and skills and began to combine them with the new knowledge they had acquired...' (Roberts *et al*, 1997, p68)

In other words, what they were describing was a manifestation of the deconstruction-reconstruction cycle as conceptualised in this text.

Figure 4.2: The inverse relationship between decontstrucion and reconstruction

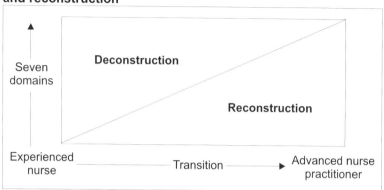

It is legitimate to question at this point whether any nurses who undertake to add new dimensions to their work role engages in the same cycle of deconstruction and reconstruction as described above. If they do not, what makes the situation of advanced practitioners different from that of any other nurse involved in role innovation? It is difficult to make generalisations when answering this question, basically because the range and extent of practice innovations taken on by nurses vary considerably. However, the evidence from this study indicates that the concept of reconstruction as it applies to advanced practitioners is clearly different from that of nurses who simply extend their role by taking on additional clinical skills and responsibilities. In the case of the latter, nurses can be seen to 'add' a limited range and number skills or activities to their practice base. However, this does not require the nurse to deconstruct any of the seven personal or practice domains to any significant degree. For example, if a nurse learns to suture minor wounds or to cannulate a patient (ie. she takes on an additional skill), while this involves minor modifications to her skill and cognitive domains, she undergoes little or no change overall in her roles, practice behaviours, identity, relationships and so on. Consequently, for the most part her role and duties remain largely unaffected, with the exception that she can now perform some additional skills. In this sense the deconstruction-reconstruction cycle is not apparent as all the nurse is doing is learning a new skill and adding it to her existing repertoire. Likewise, the cycle is equally inappropriate to describe those cases where nurses radically change their role when taking up positions such as *surgical assistants*. As suggested earlier, one could argue that the incumbent is no longer practising nursing but acting as technician and hence the notion of reconstructing nursing, can be no longer seen to apply. The fundamental difference here between ANPs and nurses such as these is that to act as a technician does not appear to involve the cycle of deconstruction and reconstruction in the sense described above. While the surgical assistant undoubtedly learns new skills and knowledge and assumes a different identity, her previous skills, knowledge, roles and identity are largely replaced or exchanged for new ones as the post demands. In other words, there is little opportunity for the nurse to integrate her existing knowledge and skills into the performance of her new work role. Hence, the role is largely one of physician assistant, which in itself, does not require any nursing qualification. Consequently, the deconstruction-reconstruction cycle as discussed in this text can be used as one method to identify nurses who undergo transition to a significantly different nursing work role from those who simply extend their skills or enter positions which are predominantly technical in nature.

Conclusion

In concluding, it is important to state that any abstract explanation that attempts to detail extremely complex cognitive processes, which in themselves cannot be readily measured, can of course be nothing more than a theorisation. This fact has been readily acknowledged in attempts to explain the concept of expertise for example (Thompson *et al*, 1990; Rolfe, 1997). It is worth re-emphasising, therefore, that the idea of the deconstruction-reconstruction cycle is an abstraction that provides another dimension to explaining some of the processes involved in the development of expert practice. In this sense, the notion of the deconstruction-reconstruction cycle is intended to complement, rather than replace, other explanations of the development of clinical expertise. The next chapter will provide a detailed explanation of the seven personal and practice domains and the way in which nursing is reconstructed during the transition of developing an advanced practice role.

References

Alex M, MacFarlane M (1992) The transition process: joint responsibility of nurse educators and employers. *Can J Nurs Admin* **5**(4):23–6

Anderson E, Leonard B, Yates J (1974) Epigenesis of the nurse practitioner role. *Am J Nurs* **74**(10):1812–16

Bass M, Rabbett P, Siskind M (1993) Novice CNS and role acquisition *Clin Nurs Spec* **7**(3):148–52

Brown M, Olshansky E (1997) From limbo to legitimacy: a theoretical model of the transition to the primary care nurse practitioner Role. *Nurs Res* **46** (1):46–51

Cameron A. (1998) *Exploring New Roles in Practice: The methodological challenge of identifying new roles.* Conference paper, Qualitative Research in Health & Social Care, Bournemouth, 30.4.98

Graham I (1991) Primary nursing: accountability is the key to its mystery. *Nurs Prac* **4**(2):26–8

Hamric A, Taylor J (1989) Role Development of the CNS. In: Hamric A,Spross J, eds *The Clinical Nurse Specialist in Theory and Practice.* 2nd edition, W. B. Saunders, Philadelphia: 41–82

Jairath N, Costello J, Wallace P, *et al* (1991) The effect of preceptorship upon diploma program nursing students' transition to the professional nursing role. *J Nurs Educ* **30**:251–5

Lukacs J (1982) Factors in nurse practitioner role adjustment. *Nurs Practitioner* March: 21, 23, 50

Meleis A (1986) Theory development and domain concepts. In: Moccia P, ed. *New Approaches to Theory Development.* National League for Nursing, New York:3–21

Murray T (1998) Using role theory concepts to understand transitions from hospital-based nursing practice to home care nursing. *J Cont Ed Nurs* **29** (3):105–11

NHS Executive (1999) Health Service Circular 1999/217, NHS Executive, London

Nicholson N (1984) A Theory of work role transitions. *Admin Science Quart* **29**:172–91

Oda D (1977) Specialized role development: a three-phase process. *Nurs Outlook* **25**(6):374–77

Roberts S, Tabloski P, Bova C (1997) Epigenesis of the nurse practitioner role revisited. *J Nurs Educ* **36**(2):67–73

Roberts-Davies M, Nolan M , Read S, *et al* (1998) Realizing specialist and advanced nursing practice: a typology of innovative nursing roles. *Acc Emerg Nurs* **6**:36–40

Rolfe G (1997) Science, abduction and the fuzzy nurse: an exploration of expertise. *J Adv Nurs* **25**:1070–75

Salussolia M (1997) Is advanced nursing practice a post or a person? *Br J Nurs* **6**(16):928, 930–3

Schumacher K, Meleis A (1994) Transitions: a central concept in nursing. *Image: J Nurs Schol.* **26**(2):119–27

Shea S, Selfridge-Thomas J (1997) The ED nurse practitioner: pearls and pitfalls of role transition and development. *J Emerg Nurs* **23**(3):235–7

Talarczyk G, Millbrandt D (1988) A collaborative effort to facilitate role transition from student to registered nurse practitioner. *Nurs Manage* **19** (2):30–2

Thompson C, Ryan S, Kitzman H (1990) Expertise: the basis for expert system development. *Adv Nurs Science* **13**:1–10

van Maanen H (1990) Nursing in transition: an analysis of the state of the art in relation to the conditions of practice and society's expectations. *J Adv Nurs* **15**:914–25

Woods L (1999) The contingent nature of advanced nursing practice. *J Adv Nurs* **30**(1):121–8

5

The seven domains of reconstruction

The seven domains of reconstruction introduced in the previous chapter will provide the focus for discussion in this one. As a reminder, these have been termed the cognition, skills, behaviour, affect, identity, relationships and roles domains. The discussion will centre on the way in which each domain develops and is reconstructed according to the orientation of role transition. A set of additional properties, which can be used to help judge the degree and extent of reconstruction within each domain, is outlined and discussed toward the end of the chapter.

Before proceeding, it is important to state at the outset that a number of studies have adopted the use of different 'domains' to explain the concept of advanced practice (Fenton, 1985; Brykczynski, 1989; Bass et al, 1993; Ackerman et al, 1996; Watts et al, 1996). Most of these studies acknowledge Benner's (1984) seminal work in identifying the seven domains of nursing practice which they have in turn taken and adapted in varying degrees for their own purposes. What each of these inquiries has in common, along with others it has to be said, is a tendency to describe advanced practice in terms of a series of roles characterised by behavioural objectives. So for example, Ackerman et al (1996) list five domains relating to acute care nurse practitioners: direct comprehensive care; support of systems; research; education; publication and professional leadership. Each domain in turn has a relevant set of behavioural indicators. The same approach appears to have been taken in the generation of the pilot standards put forward by the UKCC in its interpretation of 'a higher level of practice'. Seven discrete domains are identified, each with a unique set of standards, the majority of which are fundamentally defined in behavioural terms (NHS Executive, 1999). Many other studies have followed suit and although the domains often have different names, most conceptualise advanced practice as a series of roles with associated behavioural objectives.

While most of these studies attempt to describe the outcome (ie. the *what*) of advanced practice in terms of a series of roles, they tend to conceptualise the transitional process (or the *how*) by using Benner's (1984) novice-to-expert framework. This framework is, however, in my opinion, generally misrepresented in that it is used to describe a series of stages through which the practitioner passes at different points in time. It does little to explain the '*how*' or the '*why*' of practice reconstruction, instead conforming to the norm of identifying '*what*' a practitioner is able to achieve at the novice stage, the advanced beginner stage, the competence stage and so on.

This book takes a different approach in explaining the transitional process (ie. the *how* of becoming an advanced practitioner) by conceptualising the phenomenon of the of deconstruction-reconstruction cycle in the seven individual domains identified above. While a set of behavioural indicators could be attached to a number of these domains, for others they would be difficult to construct, for example in the case of the 'affect' and 'identity' domains. Moreover, it is argued that from the standpoint of this study, any such set of behavioural objectives would need to be defined with reference to the contingent nature of reconstruction and the influence of the social environment (Woods, 1999).

Schumacher and Meleis (1994) have identified similar concepts to those of the seven domains identified above which they prefer to call '*universal properties*'. They argue that a set of universal properties is common to most types of transition that individuals go through in life and help to differentiate transition, in all its forms, from non-transitional change. Consequently, their discussion does not specifically relate to advanced practitioners and, as a result, the way in which they define some of their universal properties differs from the way in which the seven domains of reconstruction are explained here. For example, Schumacher and Meleis (1994) fail to identify a change in the affective domain as a property of transition and, likewise, appear to amalgamate the skills and cognition domains identified above into a property they call 'abilities'. Thus, while the seven domains of reconstruction are not new concepts in themselves and have been discussed in varying combinations elsewhere, the way in which they relate to the development of a new nursing role has not been addressed explicitly by the nursing literature.

The orientation of role development

When examining the evidence from this study, one thing that became clear was that role transition ultimately involved the advanced practitioner in changing the direction or major focus of their practice in one of two ways. That is to say, that the new role *either* involved the practitioner adopting the position of 'clinician', primarily involving the delivery of direct patient care, *or* was oriented toward a position that might appropriately be described as 'orchestrator'. In the case of the latter, the practitioner becomes primarily concerned with enhancing the system of care delivery within the wider organisation. The term **consultant** could have been used to describe this orientation, however, to avoid confusion with the current debate about consultant nurses and their place in the UK healthcare system, the term orchestrator has been substituted.

The first of the two directions concerns the reconstruction of practice with the principal aim of the practitioner becoming increasingly involved in clinical activities directed toward assessment, diagnosis, treatment and management of patients, with a range of acute or chronic conditions pertaining to a specific practice discipline. The second direction of transition concerns a reconstruction of practice that is principally oriented toward enhancing the system of care delivery. In other words, practice is reconstructed so as to allow the practitioner to become primarily involved in activities that enhance the organisation and delivery of nursing care at both a ward/unit and organisational level. In the case of the latter the ANP can be considered to indirectly influence the delivery of patient care. The evidence from this inquiry does, however, suggest that ANPs may sporadically spend minimal amounts of time involved in activities characteristic of the opposing orientation of role transition, but that overall, the direction of reconstruction tends to dominate toward the extremes of the direct-indirect care practice continuum.

Subsequently, it can be asserted that it is the orientation, or focus, of the new work role which dictates to what extent each of the seven domains need to be deconstructed, and in turn determines the way in which each domain is required to be reconstructed. At the outset of the investigation the direction of transition was anticipated as being omni-directional, with what appeared to be the expectation of producing an **eclectic** practitioner able to meet a variety of practice and organisational demands (Woods, 1999). The findings of the study indicated however, that contrary to initial expectations, the orientation of practice reconstruction in *all* cases became uni-directional. That is, the orientation of practice reconstruction took one of the two directions previously identified, regardless of how the scope and boundaries of the new role were initially conceptualised and anticipated. It should be noted that this experience was associated with a sense of conflict and frustration for the ANPs who were the subject of this investigation. The implications of this will be discussed further in the following chapter.

Defining the domains

Having referred to the seven personal and practice domains on numerous occasions, this is an appropriate place to explain the phenomenon of reconstruction. For the sake of exposition the seven domains of reconstruction will be discussed discretely. However, it is important to remember that all the domains are closely inter-related, with changes in one inevitably bringing about change in one or more of the others. Moreover, the explanations that follow have been somewhat simplified so as to convey the essential features of reconstruction in a way that can be easily and widely understood. The sequence in which the domains are presented below is purely arbitrary and any conclusions drawn about the importance or otherwise of one domain over another should be set aside for the time being. The domains will be discussed in the following order; cognition, skills, behaviour, roles, affect, relationships and identity. Where appropriate, data collected during the study will be used to support the arguments presented.

Cognition

The domain of cognition relates to the changes that occur in the knowledge base and thought processes of advanced practitioners as they progress through their role transition. The first element common to this domain relates to the concept of knowledge acquisition. As would be expected of any practitioner prepared at graduate level with the aim of developing a new and advanced role, knowledge acquisition is an almost inevitable consequence of the transitional process. Indeed, in this sense, the deconstruction-reconstruction cycle discussed earlier is not immediately apparent, inasmuch as knowledge acquisition, almost by definition, means the simple 'addition' of new facts and information. To set a trend that will follow in the discussion of the other domains, it is important to point out that the study revealed that knowledge acquisition was dependent upon the orientation of role transition. As such, the advanced practitioner undergoing transition as a clinician acquired highly specialised clinical knowledge which was primarily applied to the principles of delivering direct patient care to a clearly defined client caseload. Their knowledge of anatomy, patho-physiology, diagnostic interpretation and treatment regimens for example, was greatly enhanced. The degree of advancement in this respect was clearly apparent to colleagues, as one nurse commented,

> '...I think her [ANP] knowledge base is different, on things like physiology. She's got an incredible amount of knowledge....'

The sentiment of this nurse was common to all the cases in the study, with recognition of an enhanced knowledge base being equally afforded by both nursing and medical colleagues.

For ANPs with the opposing orientation, the acquisition to their knowledge base differed somewhat. While in some cases, clinical knowledge increased, it was not to the same degree or extent as

ANPs whose role orientation was toward that of a clinician. In contrast, those ANPs whose role was oriented toward the system of care delivery demonstrated more generalised knowledge acquisition which they could apply to the various systems that influence care. In other words, their knowledge base expanded across a variety of contexts, as opposed to becoming focused on a narrow range of clinical aspects. The extent of new knowledge acquisition was nonetheless evident to the ANPs nursing and medical colleagues.

While cognitive development, particularly knowledge acquisition, was associated with the appropriation of 'propositional' knowledge gained from undertaking the master's degree programme, the cognitive changes associated with **role** development predominantly concerned the growth of 'practical knowledge', along with some affective change. For ANPs whose role was directed toward the delivery of direct care, the development of practical knowledge was evidenced over the duration of the study. The change in cognitive abilities was apparent in a number of ways, including: reduction in the supervision of clinical practice; decreasing reference to theoretical materials; increased speed in skill performance and technical procedures; and the application of skills and theoretical principles to an increasing range of patient episodes and situations. Increased cognitive ability appeared to be accompanied by affective changes, such as increases in confidence and assertiveness.

For those ANPs whose practice was of the opposite orientation, the change in cognitive ability was associated with achieving a greater breadth of knowledge. In these cases, increased practical knowledge corresponded to the nature of role acquisition. Consequently, ANPs were seen to gain 'knowledge of the system' in order to allow them to perform more effectively. Likewise, affective changes, such as increased assertiveness and confidence, accompanied cognitive and role development. These changes were frequently commented upon by case study participants as one manager pointed out,

> *'...I have seen a change in her...working relationships with people and in the way she deals with a problem ...she's much more organised in her approach to problems and problem solving....'*

Cognitive abilities were also associated with knowledge of the practice discipline and, consequently, those ANPs whose role was oriented toward staff development were still viewed as being knowledgeable about clinical issues. The following quotation illustrates the way in which cognitive and affective changes are inter-related and are perceived to be consolidated as role transition develops as ANPs come to be recognised by their peers.

'... I would say that she is more confident now, especially when she is able to argue the issues with the medics. I think she does that more confidently now.'

It is the changes in such facets as problem solving, diagnostic reasoning, decision making, as well as knowledge acquisition, that best exemplify the notion of a cycle of deconstruction and re-construction at work. It is these personal and practice attributes that the nurse has to re-define and employ in new and different ways in the performance of her new role.

Change in cognition is a well-recognised phenomenon in studies exploring the development of advanced practitioners (O'Rourke, 1989). For some reading this text, it may be apparent that I have not discussed Benner's (1984) concept of intuition in the explanation of this domain. This omission is deliberate for the reason that this work focuses on the process of role transition and how practice and the attributes of practitioners change as a result. Cognition as defined here relates primarily to changes in practical and propositional know-ledge. Undoubtedly, there is a strong argument to be made that as ANPs become more expert in their practice, they will increasingly draw on experiential knowledge as defined by Benner and others. However, there was little evidence to suggest that in the *early* stages of role transition this is the case and consequently its place in this discussion is limited.

The reconstruction of the cognition domain however, involves a lot more than simply the acquisition of new facts and information, or the development of critical thinking and problem solving skills. It is the more profound changes to this domain, along with those of the affect domain, that bring about a shift in the individual's 'world view' of what constitutes advanced nursing practice. The practitioners found this concept difficult to describe, but all vocalised that advanced practice involved, for each of them, a new way of thinking and perceiving nursing practice that intruded upon virtually every activity in which they engaged. This finding from the study clearly supports the point of view of those writers who perceive advanced practice to be defined by more than the accumulation of new skills and knowledge, or a behaviourally-based checklist of standards (Davies and Hughes, 1995; Smith, 1996; Manley, 1996).

It is evident that a substantial deconstruction and reconstruction of this domain is required to not only accommodate new information and the development of analytical skills, but is necessary in order to allow the ANPs to undergo a radical re-think of what, for many, was an established mindset and worldview of nursing.

Skills

Of the seven domains identified, it is the skills domain which has been the source of most public debate and contention. The argument goes that the acquisition of technical skills, not usually possessed by other nurses, does not, in itself, signify the presence or attainment of an advanced level of practice. This is a point of view which is difficult to dispute and is why skill acquisition is just *one* of the seven domains described here. The reason why the development of technical skills is often perceived to signify the presence of an advanced level of practice is easy to understand. The attainment of new psychomotor skills is often clearly visible to both ANP and colleagues and is perhaps the easiest aspect of role transition to explain and recognise. However, just because it is logical to conclude that the possession of additional psychomotor skills does not in itself mean a higher level of practice has been attained, it does not mean that skill acquisition as an element of advancing practice should be overlooked or trivialised.

Once again, the nature and focus of skill acquisition was found to be dependent upon the orientation of role transition. For those ANPs whose role was predominantly oriented toward the delivery of direct patient care, the acquisition of new clinical skills took priority in the early stages of role development. This was emphasised by one clinical manager, who identified,

> '... they [ANPs] had that year in university [and]...gained very little clinical experience. ... when they were coming back....they thought they were going to be involved in lots of other areas [but] one of the priorities for us on the unit was consolidation of the clinical skills.'

The ANPs initially took every opportunity to gain experience in clinical procedures and technical skills in which they were expected to become competent. Time was spent developing competence in activities such as patient assessment (along with practising the concomitant skills of inspection, palpation, percussion and auscultation); diagnostic skills; the interpretation of investigations including X-ray; and so forth. It was the possession and use of these skills that clearly distinguished the practice of ANPs from that of their nursing colleagues, who were predominantly involved in delivering what might be termed a conventional nursing service. The example of patient assessment described in the previous chapter is a good illustration of how skill acquisition fits into the deconstruction-reconstruction cycle .

For those ANPs whose role transition was oriented toward enhancing the system of care delivery, the acquisition of new skills and competencies was related to those activities required to deliver a new organisational or teaching role. Thus, gaining competence in developing practice protocols or teaching materials for example was seen to be more appropriate than learning new psychomotor skills or medical procedures. In these cases, initial attempts to acquire additional clinical skills receded as the orientation of the role became established, and ANPs acknowledged that they would be unable to develop the clinical elements of their role as initially desired. It can be seen, therefore, that changes to the skills domain is an integral part of practice development, regardless of role orientation.

Behaviour

The next domain to discuss is entitled behaviour. In this context, this domain relates to the way in which the pattern of observable behaviour of the ANP changes throughout the process of role transition. In other words, the way in which the daily activities of the ANP differ from those of nursing colleagues in terms of the changing focus of their activity. This results in changes in patterns of behaviour that are clearly observable. One feature that appeared to characterise this transition was a shift in practice priorities. This was evident in a number different ways according to whether role orientation was primarily concerned with the delivery of a service to patients, or in meeting the wider needs of the organisation. In the case of the former, the shift in focus concerned a move from delivering traditional nursing interventions, to one of comprehensive assessment and patient management. While the traditional 'caring' role was incorporated into the ANPs' practice, in these circumstances it appeared to be relegated to secondary status in the early stages of role transition. For example, the change in behaviour involved one ANP conducting a clinic in which she assessed, treated, and managed patients within a prescribed range of conditions. Undoubtedly, part of her role reflected a traditional nursing emphasis as the ANP herself points out, '... *I do believe as a nurse, I can give them a little bit more just from a counselling, advice and sympathy side of things.'*

However, she demonstrated a significant change in her pattern of behaviour as a result of the shift in practice focus. Likewise, the advanced activities in which another ANP was involved concerned the delivery of a pulmonary rehabilitation programme for both in-patients and outpatients. Once again, this required a shift in practice emphasis. The most significant shift in practice focus, however, was observed in one case where the ANP assumed a role virtually identical to that of a junior doctor in a neonatal unit. This was illustrated by the ways in which the ANP shadowed junior medical staff and worked under the supervision of the registrar on the unit upon her immediate return from the Master's programme. In this case, priority was given to gaining experience in various clinical activities such as: the examination of babies; attendance at the resuscitation neonates in the labour ward; gaining practice in invasive procedures such as umbilical arterial catheter insertion, cannulation and lumbar puncture. Consequently, the majority of the activities in which the ANP engaged were both new and novel to the role she had performed previously. It was not simply the acquisition of clinical skills that signified a change in focus [as other nurses on the unit were competent in a limited number of 'enhanced' skills, such as cannulation], but the way in which the practice behaviour of the ANP mirrored that of junior medical practitioners. In this sense, not only were the activities of the ANP similar, but the way in which her working day was organised was identical to that of junior medical staff on the unit.

ANPs whose role orientation was toward the system of care similarly altered the focus of their activity. On this occasion, the shift in focus concerned the organisational aspects of their role, such as: involvement in protocol and policy development; assessment of the need to initiate change in the practice environment; and acting as consultant or teacher to colleagues. In this way, daily patterns of behaviour differed significantly [when they were perceived to be acting in their 'advanced' role] from that of their nursing colleagues. In some instances, this took the ANP from the bedside and was seen by some to have detrimental consequences. As one junior doctor in an adult intensive care unit observed,

> '... since she started to be an advanced nurse practitioner we didn't see her in the ITU. Most of the time she is outside or in the room doing papers or preparing for things. So actually it takes her away from the ITU and again it takes her away from being in contact with the patient. And I think that the most important thing is to be in contact with the patient...'

One of the most overt aspects of changes in the behaviour domain concerned changes in practice independence and autonomy. Within the role ANPs were asked to perform, they were afforded varying degrees of practice and managerial independence and given greater autonomy in decision making. The extent of these changes was clearly apparent to the ANPs' nursing and medical colleagues as the following illustrates.

'That's the basic difference...she [ANP] doesn't have to go and ask a doctor... She can check heart and lungs, she can take the blood, she can do everything, she doesn't need to go and ask a doctor.' (Nurse manager)

'... [that] has definitely changed, she [ANP] is much more autonomous in what she does than she used to be'. (Consultant)

Corresponding to changes in practice independence and autonomy, ANPs were afforded certain privileges which were not available to other nurses. When the role involved the delivery of direct care, these included such things as: ordering expensive investigations independently; altering treatment regimens; admitting patients without medical approval; and in one instance moderate prescription privileges via protocol. Consequently, the data revealed that while the ANPs had very little discretion to adjust the boundaries and scope of their new role, they were afforded a higher degree of discretion and practice independence **within** the context of care delivery.

Likewise for those ANPs who had a primarily organisational role, increased independence was associated with privileges such as: freedom of time management; the autonomy to amend protocols and educational programmes as considered necessary; and the freedom of access to resources and personnel. In this respect, increased autonomy and independence can be considered to be a common feature of role development, regardless of role orientation, and is clearly observable in the way in which patterns of behaviour change. When the role is oriented to that of clinician, patterns of behaviour change so as to facilitate practice independence, whereas in the opposing orientation, managerial independence is more evident.

While discussing this domain, it is appropriate to briefly address the attribute of leadership recognised as an essential characteristic of advanced practitioners (Jackson, 1995; O'Flynn, 1996). Interestingly, in this study leadership behaviours were not immediately observable in the day-to-day practice of ANPs. One manager who was interviewed made it clear that leadership behaviours were not anticipated to be present in the early stages of role transition,

'...we're just not seeing any evidence of leadership from the introduction of this role. [The ANP] ... is just concentrating on developing her new skills and getting the new components

of her role sorted out. Perhaps, hopefully, in the future we will see more evidence of leadership, but at the moment, that's not the case.'

It appears then from the findings of this study, that in at least the early stages of role development, practitioners are pre-occupied with skill acquisition and role clarification. Consequently, the attribute of leadership, as discussed in the advanced practitioner literature, appears to be subjugated in the initial period of role transition. Of course, one could argue that the development of the roles and functions that are associated with advanced practice are in and of themselves evidence of nursing leadership. The problem of this position becomes one of how 'leadership' is perceived, understood and recognised between different stakeholders. If one adopts a view that leadership is fundamentally about empowering and influencing other nurses (O'Flynn, 1996) both directly and indirectly, to progress practice, then those ANPs whose orientation is toward the system of care delivery are likely to be in a stronger position to demonstrate leadership characteristics. However, leadership is also about taking personal risks, breaking practice boundaries, and having insight and vision into perceiving new ways of delivering care, not simply from an organisational context, but from the perspective of the individual practitioner. In this instance, those ANPs whose roles focus primarily on the delivery of nursing care as advanced clinicians are in prime positions to take nursing forward. The issue of leadership then becomes one of perspective, which is not easily reconciled. However, Jackson (1995) warns that practitioners must develop competence as leaders [as well as in other domains] if they are to be *recognised* as advanced practice nurses. Perhaps it is more realistic to acknowledge that,

'... the sheer amount of information and knowledge needed for advanced practice may be overwhelming ... Therefore, rather than trying to know everything by graduation, a recognition of self as a life-long learner is essential.' (O'Flynn, 1996)

This notion could apply not only to practical competencies and skills, but also to characteristics and traits such as leadership, confidence and so on. As with other skills and attributes, leadership qualities may emerge over time as the practitioners become established and comfortable within their roles. It is sufficient to say however, that in the context of this study, that there was insufficient evidence to suggest that leadership qualities were developed as a *consequence* of role transition. Some ANPs certainly exhibited more leadership characteristics than others, but this appeared to be defined more by the type of personality and past experiences of the individuals concerned, as opposed to being directly attributable to the transitional process in which ANPs engaged.

Roles

The next domain concerns the new roles that advanced practitioners take on as a consequence of their transition. In a general sense, the move from experienced nurse to that of advanced practitioner represents a significant change in role in itself. However, the concept of role as it is applies to the seven domains of reconstruction is somewhat different. As a concept, it is more akin to that discussed in the context of the North American literature concerning advanced practitioners. As was outlined in *Chapter 1* many writers explain the nature of advanced practice in terms of a series of sub-roles such as, clinician, educator, researcher, administrator and consultant. While there appears to be a general consensus that advanced practitioners in North America accommodate each of these sub-roles in varying degrees, similar assertions of advanced practitioners in the UK remain largely unsubstantiated. With this in mind, this study sought to establish if the sub-roles of advanced practitioners as outlined in the North American literature were exhibited by UK nurses undergoing transition to become advanced practitioners.

As with a number of other domains discussed in this chapter, the answer to this question was related to the orientation of role transition. However, over the duration of this investigation, none of the practitioners involved in the study managed to advance their practice in *all* of the sub-roles identified in the literature. In effect, the notion of an advanced practitioner with an eclectic role orientation, able to demonstrate competence over a wide range of activities, failed to emerge. Of course, this could have been due to a number of factors such as the early stage in role development, the small sample of practitioners involved in the study and the constraints imposed by key stakeholders within the employing organisation. Indeed, the evidence from the study revealed that the latter played a significant part in stifling the development of an eclectic role that many stakeholders idealised at the outset of the transitional process (Woods, 1999). It is also important to acknowledge that when talking of the sub-roles adopted by practitioners these are not simply replications of roles they undertook as experienced nurses. In other words, *any* nurse could argue that they fulfilled, at least to some extent, each of the sub-roles identified above. What is important to remember is that each of these sub-roles, while still maintaining a nursing focus, is likely to be enacted at a more complex and comprehensive level by the advanced practitioner, and consequently differ considerably. So was this case in this study?

For those practitioners whose overall role took the orientation of clinician, the sub-role of 'clinician', perhaps to state the obvious, was clearly evident. That is, the ANPs focused on fulfilling clinical responsibilities. Thus for example, one ANP independently ran an early pregnancy assessment clinic where she would assess, examine, and determine the patient's trajectory, which resulted in either admission, discharge, booking for theatre or the provision of counselling and support. In another case, the ANP would, on request, attend mothers in the labour suite and perform the resuscitation of neonates, arrange for admission, examine the baby and perform the necessary therapeutic interventions. These roles were clearly enacted at a more complex and comprehensive level than by other nurses within the organisation and had a substantively different focus. However, due to the contingent nature of advanced practice and the constraints placed on ANPs by key stakeholders in the organisation, along with limited resources, ANPs failed to make significant progress in the development of other sub-roles. For example, the sub-role of consultant was primarily drawn upon from the point of view of the ANP's *clinical* knowledge and skills. Consequently, consultancy rarely, if at all, concerned organisational issues or matters of policy. Likewise, in the other sub-roles, ANPs had only limited opportunity to consolidate the skills and experience necessary for them to add new dimensions to their practice.

For practitioners whose role took an opposing orientation the reverse was evident. When the role was aimed towards enhancing the system of care delivery and the organisation, there was progress in some sub-roles at the expense of others. In this case, it was the role of clinician that failed to progress. At the end of the study, those ANPs whose role followed this orientation admitted that the direct patient care they delivered was predominantly similar in nature to that of their experienced nursing colleagues. Consequently, the 'clinical' role they enacted was at no more a complex or comprehensive level than other nurses' within the organisation and had a substantively similar focus. Development in the sub-roles of educator and administrator, along with that of consultant, were however, clearly evident. For example, in one case, an ANP in an accident and emergency department became responsible for developing and delivering an emergency nurse practitioner (ENP) programme. The course was previously delivered predominantly by medical staff, who were also responsible for supervising the practice of ENPs. The ANP in this case not only took over the teaching of a number of the sessions previously delivered by medical staff, but was also responsible for supervising ENPs in clinical practice and even getting the programme accredited with the local university. In another case, an ANP took a lead on practice protocol development at an organisational level. She was called upon to provide consultancy about practice and policy by a number of other units and wards throughout the hospital. In this instance, the ANP's managerial and administrative sub-roles were enacted at a more complex and comprehensive level than by other nurses within the organisation and once again had a substantively different focus.

It may not have escaped the more observant, that no reference to the sub-role of researcher has yet been made. There was an initial expectation by all those interviewed at the outset of the study that ANPs would take a lead in facilitating the utilisation of research findings and implementation of evidence-based practice by nursing colleagues. In addition, in the majority of cases there was an expectation that ANPs would develop research proposals and undertake empirical studies appropriate to their area of practice. By the end of the study, in all the cases, this was the one sub-role in which little or no development was evident. For most, lack of time and resources was given as the reason for failing to develop this activity. However, there are obvious similarities with ANPs in the UK and their counterparts in other countries with regard to this phenomenon. There is some corroborating evidence that advanced practitioners appear to spend very little time undertaking activities associated with this sub-role (Cooper and Sparacino, 1990). Arguably, another reason why ANPs may not have developed this sub-role is that, in essence, research is seen as a luxury and consequently is given only lip-service with the result that it comes low down in the practice priorities of many practitioners.

In summary, the roles that ANPs develop are related to the orientation of their transition with the result that when the role is primarily that of 'clinician', clinical roles and responsibilities predominate. For those ANPs with an opposing orientation, organisational roles and responsibilities predominate.

Affect

The next domain to discuss concerns affect, or in other words, the attitudinal and value changes that accompany role transition. This domain differs somewhat from those detailed above, in that, to some extent, it is not as easy to recognise as changes in roles, skills or behaviour that accompany role transition. It is, nonetheless, another domain that undergoes transformation according to the general orientation that the transition takes. Two specific examples may best serve to illustrate the change in the affective domain.

The nursing literature is replete with accounts of how patient care has been *medicalised* by doctors, with the accusation being that the majority exhibit a reductionist approach to patient management. The typical view held by nurses is one of the medical profession relating to patients by way of their symptoms or medical condition, eg. the 'kidney in bed 3' phenomenon. Nursing on the other hand in recent years has purportedly rejected this approach in favour of 'holism' and 'individualism', characterised by nurses relating to patients as people, eg. the 'person in bed 3' approach. Each of these strategies has an associated value system characterised respectively by the concepts of *cure* and *care*. When advanced practitioners are involved in role transition which is oriented toward the delivery of direct patient care, they engage in the deconstruction of their attitudes and value system in order to accommodate the roles, skills and activities that their new position demands. In this case a number of the practices in which they are expected to become competent are more commonly associated with the practice of medicine. What is reconstructed then is an affective domain that still regards the concepts of holism and individualism as central, but increasingly becomes accepting of the medical needs of the patient and the need to treat the symptoms, as well as the person. Likewise, when the direction of role transition is toward enhancing the system of care delivery, the values of the practitioner in terms of seeing herself and her immediate priorities uppermost, are reconstructed so as to acknowledge and react to the needs of the organisational system within which she works. Hence, whereas in the past the practitioner would be quick to blame the 'system', she now acknowledges and recognises its bureaucratic idiosyncrasies and may even make excuses for it.

There are of course many other ways in which the affective domain changes. Some of these are subtle while others, such as those examples described above, are more apparent. It should not be forgotten that changes in this domain, along with those in the cognitive domain, are responsible for the major shifts that occur in the worldview of individual practitioners. Consequently, it is the changes that occur in this area which are some of the most profound. Ironically, they are also some of the changes that are the most difficult to uncover and observe.

Relationships

The penultimate domain to discuss in relation to the transitional process pertains to the relationships that ANPs have to reconstruct with both their nursing and medical colleagues. It should be no surprise by now that, once again, the nature of reconstruction appears to be dependent upon the overall orientation of the role. The data from the study revealed that ANPs deconstruct their prior relationships in order to form new ones which are necessary for role enactment. Thus, when the direction of role transition is toward the delivery of direct care, the ANP reconstructs her relationships predominantly with physicians, whereas for the ANP with an opposing orientation, the reconstruction of relationships is with her nursing colleagues.

It is important to note that in this study, the majority of ANPs were not deployed in a full-time supernumerary capacity following their educational preparation to take on the role as advanced practitioner. In such cases, individuals experienced role dualism, inasmuch as for half of the time they were expected to develop an advanced practice role and take on new responsibilities, whereas at other times, they were required to take on their old role, duties and responsibilities so as to meet immediate organisational needs. Consequently, when they were acting in their old role they were treated in a similar fashion to other nurses. The ANP's own perceptions were that they were viewed with little difference by the majority of the nursing staff with whom they worked when acting in such a capacity. However, when the ANPs formally adopted their advanced role and attempted to develop their practice in new ways, relationships were clearly different.

Following a one year absence from the work place [as a result of the full-time master's programme], ANPs were required to re-negotiate relationships upon their return to work. It appeared that relationships with managers proved most problematic, although some experienced difficulties with senior medical colleagues. For those ANPs whose role overlapped considerably with that of medical colleagues, difficulties were experienced not only with junior doctors, but also with some nursing colleagues. It is interesting to observe that, despite the perceived minimal change in relationships with nursing peers when undertaking a traditional nursing role, when ANPs were afforded time to spend in practice development, they appeared to experience a change in status. When this occurred, ANPs were both perceived and treated differently from other nursing staff. Interestingly, this was manifest most overtly in the way in which ANPs experienced conflict with their nursing colleagues, concerning both the philosophy and practice orientation of their new role. From a philosophical standpoint, some ANPs were seen by a few of their colleagues to be selling out traditional nursing values. As one nurse manager noted, the ANPs found,

> '... it quite difficult when they came back because they seemed to have no impact into nursing. Because the medical supervisors had them looking at almost, training them as they would a junior intensivist...nurses resented that a lot. What's that to do with nursing?'

In this case, in order to fulfil the clinical requirements of the new role, and to achieve some degree of practice independence and respect of her medical colleagues, the ANP attempted to deconstruct the hierarchical relationships that previously existed. This entailed a number of strategies and changes in patterns of behaviour described earlier. An important feature of re-negotiating relationships with professional colleagues and in gaining legitimation for the new role concerned establishing clinical credibility. This concept varied according to the way in which the new role was being developed. In cases where the ANP was primarily involved in delivering patient care, clinical credibility was chiefly associated with gaining competence in psychomotor skills, clinical procedures and tasks. In such cases, the standard of practice was compared with that of medical practitioners, as few, if any other nurses were performing the same roles or skills. Of course, as an inevitable consequence of role transition, relationships with nursing colleagues did alter, but not to the same extent as those with medical colleagues. ANPs openly negotiated the parameters of their role development with nursing managers, but more so with senior medical staff, to whom a number were accountable clinically. Interestingly, just as Conway (1996) found in her study of nursing experts it was the ANPs who adopted a more proactive and flexible stategy when re-negotiating relationships with their medical colleagues.

For ANPs whose role orientation was directed toward the system of care delivery, the change in relationships with medical colleagues was less evident. While there may have been increased contact with senior medical staff concerning the nature of their role development, the general nature of the relationship remained largely unaltered. On the other hand, it was the relationships with nursing colleagues which ANPs were required to reconstruct. In these cases, as the new role did not involve the ANP in acting in a medical replacement capacity, the difficulties experienced with nursing colleagues were related to the impact of the new role on senior managers. Conflict appeared to be associated with the perceived threat the ANP posed to managers' existing roles. However, once the ANPs had become established in their new roles, the incidence of conflict with nursing colleagues and nursing managers receded. Once again the issue of credibility emerged as being an important feature in the re-construction of relationships. In cases where the ANP role was oriented toward the system of care delivery credibility in maintaining traditional nursing skills was seen to be of prime importance. As one manager noted,

> '...the views of all the senior nurses is ... that for them to maintain their roles as ANPs they've got to be seen clinically out there doing the job. They've got to be clinically credible.'

Clinical credibility in this context was primarily associated with general nursing care activities (as opposed to any advanced activities) and the need for the ANP to act as a role model to other nursing staff while engaged in practice. This may provide one explanation why some managers appear actively to control the limits of role development.

For ANPs whose role primarily involved education, administration and consultancy, a change in relationships with nursing colleagues was required in order to achieve credibility in the new role. One nurse commented that she no longer viewed her ANP colleague as a peer, but akin to a manager. This comment probably explains both how and why ANPs who take on such a role have to reconstruct their relationships predominantly with nursing colleagues, while only seeing moderate changes in relationships with medical colleagues.

Identity

The final domain concerns the notion of professional identity. Unlike all the other domains, this is the only exception to the rule of dichotomy, inasmuch as all the ANPs in the study appeared to occupy the same position on the continuum. The evidence from the study indicates that ANPs expressly sought to gain recognition for their practice development. This can be considered to be the first stage in the establishment of a new and different professional identity. It has previously been recognised that individuals can undergo a radical change in personal identity following movement into a new work role or situation (Van Maanen and Schein, 1979). However, in the context of this study, the ANPs' desire to change their identities has implications for the professional basis of nursing and thus goes beyond the simple change in personal identity that appears to accompany any transition (Schumacher and Meleis, 1994). It is asserted here that, regardless of the operational outcome of role transition, the ANPs' determination to seek recognition and to establish new identities remains constant. In other words, whether the outcome of practice reconstruction was oriented toward clinical practice or the system of care, the ANPs still sought to have their new professional identities acknowledged and recognised by others.

In the process of seeking to establish themselves as practitioners with unique identities, ANPs appeared to experience a conflict in their own 'nursing' identities. This was most noticeable in those for whom the process of role transition was problematic. The origin of their conflict was associated with disenchantment with the traditional nursing roles in which they were required to engage during the transition. This led to a paradox whereby, while ANPs espoused the virtues of nursing and its underpinning philosophy, each sought to distance themselves from that traditional identity in order to be recognised in their new capacity. That is not to suggest that ANPs intentionally devalued nursing or their nursing colleagues, merely that in the context of their development they associated themselves with a different identity. In so doing, most appeared to suppress their nursing identity in favour of seeking recognition as advanced practitioners. The notion of practitioners submerging their nursing identity is not new. Studies have found that *during* educational preparation for advanced practice, nurses have experienced a temporary loss of identity and skills as a consequence of having to learn new skills and theory more commonly associated with the practice of medicine (Anderson *et al*, 1974; Roberts *et al*, 1997). The importance of the change in identity is such, that it will be discussed extensively in the next chapter.

Figure 5.1 illustrates the relationship of each domain to the orientation of role transition and their dichotomous nature.

Figure 5.1: The seven domains of reconstruction

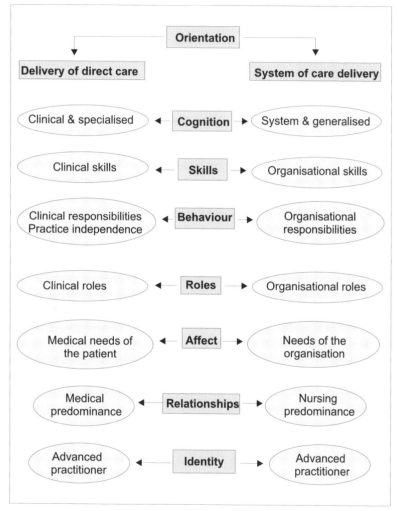

Properties

Each of the seven domains of reconstruction described above can be considered to have a set of properties. These properties relate to the concepts of magnitude; scope; rate; and context. By utilising certain of these domain properties one is able to establish not only in what ways practice has been reconstructed, but how quickly, and to what extent. Taken together, they give an indication of whether the practitioner has achieved an advanced stage of practice in comparison to other nurses within the clinical setting, or has only made minor modifications to their role.

The first property, magnitude, relates to the extent of change within each domain. So for example, where there are only small degrees of change within each domain one could conclude that reconstruction has either not occurred or at best has been conservative. Correspondingly, the greater the degree of change within each domain the more radical the role transition and the more noticeable the change in nursing practice.

The second property, scope, is obviously related to the overall orientation of role transition that has already been discussed. As is evident, the scope of change in each domain can be correspondingly broad or narrow. The evidence would seem to suggest that the wider the scope of reconstruction, the more eclectic the role orientation is likely to become and the more likely the practitioner is to develop the whole sphere of advanced nursing practice. In contrast, the narrower the scope of reconstruction, the more likely that practice will develop along uni-dimensional lines. In other words, rather than advancing practice from a generalist or eclectic perspective, it is more likely that the subsequent role will become highly specialised and focused in one particular direction.

The third property, rate, concerns the pace of reconstruction within each domain and in this respect is closely associated with the nature of the contingent conditions within the practice setting. Subsequently, if conditions are favourable, the pace of reconstruction can be sustained at a constant rate. If on the other hand, contingent conditions are volatile and disabling, then the pace of reconstruction becomes sporadic with the overall rate progress being delayed.

The final property, context, locates dimensional changes in each domain to the demands of the local environment. In turn this has implications for the transferability of the ANPs' roles and skills to other practice settings. The evidence from this study indicates that for advanced practitioners in acute care settings, the more extensively they engage in practice reconstruction, the more context-specific it becomes. The influence of the practice specialism, the orientation of role transition, the level of patient dependency, and the contingent nature of reconstruction each dictate that the expertise the practitioner develops during role transition is highly individualised. It is for these reasons that expertise is seen to be non-transferable and is consistent with Alspach's (1984) assertion that when competency is demonstrated in relation to a specific field, setting, role or level of practice, the alteration of any of these elements undermines the competency of the practitioner. So for example, whereas nurses are generally able to move relatively freely between different specialities during their career, if an advanced practitioner were to move to a completely different clinical speciality (which is obviously unlikely), she would, at least in the short-term, no longer be considered to be advanced in her practice. A similar conclusion was reached following a series of interviews conducted by Fulbrook (1998) whereby ANPs acknowledged a core of advanced practice that had utility regardless of context, but conceded that advanced practice was located in a specific field of clinical practice. However, although ANPs are unlikely to move between disciplines, they may possibly move between practice settings within the same discipline. Dillon and George's (1997) UK study found that ANPs working in different neonatal units performed broadly the same function and skills, which demonstrates that within- discipline mobility will not necessarily be restricted. The same is probably true for other specialisms.

Conclusion

In a relatively limited amount of space this chapter has attempted to convey the fundamental changes that take place during the transition of moving from an established, experienced nurse, to that of a neophyte advanced practitioner. It has proposed that by examining the changes that take place in seven individual and practice domains, account can be taken of not only how the practice of ANPs differs from that of their colleagues, but what is involved in the transitional process. Conceivably, it is possible for each of the domains described above to be considered in isolation and to plot, or at least try to plot, the degree and extent of change along each domain continuum. In attempting to measure the extent of role transition however, it is recommended that the seven domains be considered in relationship with one another and not be treated individually. This is because it is suggested that, only when changes to each domain have been maximised within the context of the clinical setting, a level of advanced practice can be considered to have been attained. In other words, a practitioner cannot be considered to have reached an advanced level of practice if, for example, he/she has only maximised reconstruction of his/her skill base, while exhibiting minimal changes in the other domains. On the other hand, somebody who exhibits major changes to his/her cognitive abilities, skills, relationships, roles, values, behaviours and identity, clearly can be seen to have attained a different practice status when compared to his/her nursing peers in the same setting. It is, therefore, the overall profile of the practitioner in terms of the level of development of each of the seven domains which provides the clearest indication that a state of advanced practice has been achieved.

As mentioned in *Chapter 1*, the personal attributes of the practitioner undoubtedly have a significant impact on the way in which the role transition is managed and experienced. Moreover, there are many changes that are difficult to quantify and evaluate, such as the change in the worldview of advanced practice that accompanies transition, affective changes, cognitive processes and so on. While acknowledging the individual characteristics of practitioners and the complex and individualised nature of personal and role changes, this chapter has, nonetheless, attempted to generate a model of transition which can be applied to a wide variety of advanced practice roles and contexts. When this framework is used to examine the outcome of role transition as a whole, the indication is that when the new role is oriented toward the delivery of direct care, many of the practice characteristics of the ANP are consistent with the role of the 'nurse practitioner' as described in the North American literature. Likewise, when practice reconstruction is oriented toward the system of care delivery it shares many of the similarities that are present in the practice of 'clinical nurse specialists' as described in the North American literature (for example, see Fenton and Brykczynski, 1993). Both of these established roles are well founded and recognised to be advanced in nature in the international literature (Autar, 1996). I am not suggesting that ANPs in the UK necessarily adopt these titles, although some have already done so, I merely observe that many similarities between such roles exist.

The final chapter will examine the various outcomes of the transitional process that were found to occur amongst the ANPs in this study and compare them with those described in the literature.

References

Ackerman M, Norsen L, Martin B *et al* (1996) Development of a model of advanced practice *Am J Crit Care* **5**(1):68–73

Alspach J (1984) Designing a competency-based orientation for critical care nurses. *Heart Lung* **13**:655–62

Anderson E, Leonard B, Yates J (1974) Epigenesis of the nurse practitioner role. *Am J Nurs.* **74**(10):1812–16

Autar R (1996) Role of the nurse teacher in advanced nursing practice. *Br J Nurs* **5**(5):298–301

Bass M, Rabbett P, Siskind M (1993) Novice CNS and role acquisition *Clin Nurs Spec* **7**(3):148–52

Benner P (1984) *From Novice to Expert*. Addison-Wesley, London

Brykczynski K (1989) An interpretive study describing the clinical judgement of nurse practitioners. *Schol Inq Nurs Pract.* **3**(2):75–104

Conway J (1996) *Nursing Expertise and Advanced Practice*. Quay Bookes, Mark Allen Publishing Ltd, Dinton, Wilts

Cooper D, Sparacino P (1990) Acquiring, implementing and evaluating the clinical nurse specialist role. In: Sparacino P, Cooper D, Minarik P, eds. *The Clinical Nurse Specialist: Implementation and Impact*. Appleton and Lange, Norwalk, Connecticut: 41–75

Davies B, Hughes A (1995) Clarification of advanced nursing practice: Characteristics and competencies. *Clin Nurs Spec* **9**(3):156–60

Dillon A, George S (1997) Advanced neonatal nurse practitioners in the United Kingdom: where are they and what do they do? *J Adv Nurs* **25**: 257–64

Fenton M (1985) Identifying competencies of clinical nurse specialists. *J Nurs Admin* **15**(12):31–7

Fenton M, Brykczynski K (1993) Qualitative Distinctions and Similarities in the Practice of Clinical Nurse Specialists and Nurse Practitioners. *J Profl Nurs* **9**(6):313–26

Fulbrook P (1998) Advanced practice: the 'advanced practitioner' perspective. In: Rolfe G, Fulbrook P, eds. *Advanced Nursing Practice*. Butterworth-Heinemann, Oxford:87–102

Jackson P (1995) Advanced practice nursing part 2 — opportunities and challenges for PNPs. *Ped Nurs.* **21**(1):43–6

Manley K (1996) Advanced practice is not about medicalising nursing roles *Nurs Crit Care* **1**(2):56–7

NHS Executive (1999) Health Service Circular 1999/217, NHS Executive, London

O'Flynn A (1996) The preparation of advanced practice nurses. *Nurs Clin North Am* **31**(3):429–38

O'Rourke M (1989) Generic professional behaviours: Implications for the Clinical Nurse Specialist Role. *Clin Nurs Spec* 3(2):128–32

Roberts S, Tabloski P, Bova C (1997) Epigenesis of the nurse practitioner role revisited. *J Nurs Educ* **36**(2):67–3

Schumacher K, Meleis A (1994) Transitions: a central concept in nursing. *Image: J Nurs Schol* **26**(2):119–27

Smith S (1996) Independent nurse practitioner. *Nurs Clin North Am* **31** (3):549–63

van Maanen J, Schein E (1979) Toward a theory of organisational socialization. In: Staw B, ed. *Research in organisational behaviour, Vol 1*. JAI Press, Greenwich, CT: 209–64

Watts R, Hanson M, Burke K *et al* (1996) The critical care nurse practitioner: an advanced practice role for the critical care nurse. *Dim Crit Care Nurs* **15**(1):48–56

Woods L (1999) The contingent nature of advanced nursing practice. *J Adv Nurs* **30**(1):121–8

6

The outcomes of role transition

This chapter examines the outcomes of practice reconstruction. The following discussion takes account of not only the early stage in the evolution of the ANP role in the UK, but also the limitations associated with the brevity of this study. The following commentary explores the study's findings regarding the outcomes of role transition, as well as considering the future impact of the continuing development of the advanced nurse practitioner role. To date, the discussion has illustrated the different ways in which practice is reconstructed when the orientation of role transition is focused toward either the delivery of direct care, or the system of care delivery. Furthermore, the contingent nature of role transition has been highlighted to illustrate how the process and outcome of role transition are influenced by a variety of factors in the social setting (Woods, 1999). The following argument develops a simple classification of role transition outcomes and demonstrates their relationship to the contingent conditions and the properties associated with the seven domains of reconstruction. It will be contested that the outcomes of practice reconstruction can be considered to exist on two conceptual levels. The first, which has been termed the 'operational outcome', relates to a concept of practice reconstruction which to a large extent is observable in the roles, behaviours, skills and relationships of the advanced practitioner. The second, and arguably more subtle outcome, concerns the beginnings of a change in professional identity associated with the role transition from experienced nurse to advanced nurse practitioner. The chapter concludes by addressing the implications for the establishment of a new professional identity for both practitioners and the nursing profession as a whole.

Following analysis and consideration of the data collected in this study, three operational outcomes of practice reconstruction were eventually developed: practice replication; practice fragmentation; and practice innovation. These outcomes were adapted from Nicholson's (1984) *Theory of Work Role Transition*. It is not intended to discuss Nicholson's theory in any depth here and those wishing to read more about it are referred to the original text which gives a comprehensive account of its development and characteristics. However, it is pertinent to state that while Nicholson's (1984) theory was posited over a decade ago, it has been utilised in a number of recent studies to explore the phenomenon of work role transition (see: Black and Ashford, 1995; Glen and Waddington, 1998). The results of these, and other studies, have found varying degrees of support for the theory and while some suggest modifications to the framework, the fundamental propositions of the theory have not been significantly challenged.

When Nicholson's (1984) theory was first developed, it was intended for use as a 'grand' theory to enable prediction of the outcome of work role transitions in a wide variety and types of organisations. The desire to refine and adapt the theory for the purpose of this study was based on the wish to apply an appropriate theoretical framework and its principles to the phenomenon of increasing numbers of nurses undergoing work role transitions. In addition, the need to develop a conceptual framework in which account could be taken of the unique characteristics and organisational structures in which nurses are employed became equally apparent.

Practice replication

The first operational outcome of practice reconstruction to be addressed relates to its concept. This outcome shares many conceptual similarities with Nicholson's (1984) idea of replication as one potential mode of adjustment in work role transition. He describes replication as,

> '...those transitions that generate minimal adjustment to personal or role systems. The new incumbent makes few adjustments in ... her role identity or behaviour to fit into the new role and makes no changes in role requirements. The person performs in much the same manner as in previous jobs and also in much the same manner as previous occupants.' (Nicholson, 1984, pp175–76).

Replication in this case can be seen to be characterised by low degrees of personal and role development. Consequently, the individual encounters low levels of novelty in practice. In the context of this investigation, for whatever reason, practitioners fail to develop 'new' clinical skills or experience new and novel ways of organising and delivering nursing care. At the same time individuals have little or no discretion to control the orientation or scope of practice development. The result is a minimal change in the work role and hence the evidence of an advanced level of practice is not readily apparent. Nicholson (1984) argues that when (practice) replication occurs, personal development is low. He argues that there is little personal change in identity, abilities, skills, values or frame of reference. While this may be accurate for individuals moving between established jobs, the evidence from this study suggests a contrary position where the role is **new** to an organisation and the individual. In the case of ANPs, undergoing the transition required formal academic preparation at the master's degree level, which in turn inevitably resulted in some degree of personal development. In the one case study where practice replication was the outcome, the ANP experienced a change in identity, values and frame of reference. Moreover, while there were only minimal changes in her psychomotor and clinical skills, cognitive development was acknowledged to have taken place. Consequently, in contrast to Nicholson's (1984) theory, it is argued that in this set of circumstances, personal development can be seen to occur. Thus, low personal development may be identified as a key variable by Nicholson (1984) to explain the replication mode of adjustment to a new work role, but in the context of this study the evidence indicates a somewhat contrary point of view.

On the other hand, Nicholson's (1984) articulation of the concept of **role** development and its association with the corresponding modes of adjustment is more consistent with the findings of this study. Nicholson (1984) argued that replication results when there is little change to the parameters or requirements of the work role and the person performs in much the same manner as in previous jobs. The evidence from this inquiry clearly indicates that one ANP performed in much the same way following preparation for the new role as she did prior to entering the transitional process (ie. practice was replicated). Consequently, role development in the sense of *'...changes in task objectives, methods, materials, scheduling, and interpersonal relationships integral to role performance'* (Nicholson, 1984, p175), can be considered to have been low. It is important to state that the underpinning reasons for this outcome are clearly linked to organisational constraints and the contingent nature of advanced practice, and not to the inability or desires of the individual practitioner. Nicholson (1984) acknowledges that,

> *'Role development varies according to the constraints and opportunities of the role and the needs and expectations of the person.'* (p175)

However, he appears to underestimate the influence that contingent conditions may exert on the transitional process.

Nicholson (1984) identifies two further key variables that have a major influence on the nature of work role transitions: novelty and discretion. According to Nicholson's (1984) theory, novelty is associated with the degree to which prior knowledge, skills, and activities can be utilised in the performance of the new work role and is also identified with personal development. Low levels of novelty are associated with the concept of 'replication' in that the individual primarily utilises existing knowledge and skills in the performance of the new work role. In the context of this study, 'practice replication' conforms to this notion, as one ANP acknowledged, '*... it's not really that new at all. Some bits are, but a lot of it is what I was already doing before'.*

However, the fact that the ANP was experiencing low levels of novelty in her role was due to the contingent conditions which were preventing her from developing new and novel practices. When utilising novelty as a predictor variable then, one needs to be cognisant of the nature and influence of contingent conditions.

The final key variable to consider in relation to practice replication is Nicholson's (1984) concept of discretion. This concept needs to be considered as a multi-dimensional construct, which in this book is identified as comprising **organisational** as well as **within-role** discretion. The degree of discretion afforded the individual when practice replication is the resultant outcome of transition varies along each dimension. That is to say the individual can have high levels of within-role discretion, but low levels of discretion to move outside the parameters of the new work role as it had been constructed under the aegis of organisational governance (Woods, 1999). Discretion can be more readily utilised as a predictor variable when measured in conjunction with the degree of role development experienced by an individual.

The relationship between Nicholson's (1984) four key variables and the outcome of role transition classified as practice replication is illustrated in *Table 6.1*.

Table 6.1: Relationship between practice replication and key variables				
Outcome/ variable>	Role development	Personal development	Novelty	Discretion
Practice replication	Low	Moderate	Low	Low*- moderate/high#
*=Organisational discretion; #=within-role discretion				

This outcome would suggest that the transition from experienced nurse to advanced nurse practitioner has to a large degree failed to succeed. This conclusion is based on the observation that little of what the ANP role involves in terms of activities, roles, responsibilities and so on can be considered to be new, novel or different from the way in which the ANP was practising prior to entering the transitional process. As a word of warning, the utilisation of the key indicators identified above can be of limited value if the practitioner has already achieved an advanced level practice *prior* to engaging in formal role transition. In other words, if someone, for whatever reason, and by whatever means, has developed their practice to an advanced level *before* undergoing formal training, changes in novelty, discretion and so on, may not necessarily be detected following the transition. This does not mean to say however, that they have failed to demonstrate an advanced level of practice. Indeed, this was the case in this study. Therefore, while the likelihood of such cases is probably going to be limited, the criteria discussed in this chapter need to be utilised carefully to avoid reaching the wrong conclusions.

Practice innovation

The outcome of role transition at the opposite end of the continuum from practice replication has been termed 'practice innovation'. Practice innovation has been used to replace Nicholson's (1984) corresponding mode of adjustment which he referred to as 'exploration'. The change in terminology identifies the concept as one that is more commonly used and understood in practice-based disciplines. For Nicholson (1984), exploration is the mode of adjustment that relates to simultaneous changes in role parameters and personal qualities affecting the outcome of work role transition. In the context of this inquiry, practice innovation is defined as the reconstruction of practice parameters requiring the development of new skills and activities and which results in increased practice independence and autonomy, as well as changes in personal qualities. Utilising the four variables associated with work role transitions it is possible to illustrate the essential differences between practice innovation and the outcome of practice replication discussed earlier.

The first variable, role development, is the single most important indicator that practice innovation has occurred. Moreover, the more extensive the degree of role development the more radical the nature of practice innovation. That is to say, that when the transition involves the practitioner engaging in largely new and novel practices, designed to enhance and benefit the delivery of nursing care both directly and indirectly, then practice innovation can be seen to have occurred. By its very nature, role development in this context, which involves a considerable change in practice parameters and activities, inevitably leads to a high degree of personal development. This is because not only is the ANP required to develop and learn new skills and knowledge, but is also required to undergo a change in practice values. Sometimes however, this 'new' set of values may be dissonant with the ANP's existing nursing values, dependent upon the nature of the role transition. That is, the effect of contingent conditions may result in the practitioner developing her role in radically new ways which may be at odds with her own values of how advanced practice should be developed.

The third variable, novelty, is also by the nature of practice innovation experienced to a high degree for the reasons explained above. Likewise, with regard to the final variable, discretion, when the outcome of role transition is practice innovation, ANPs experience a substantial change in the amount of discretion that they are afforded **within** their role (when compared to other nurses or measured against their old role). Yet again however, the ANP can experience little discretion to move outside the parameters of practice reconstruction as they have been determined and consequently, just as with practice replication, organisational governance can be seen to regulate the degree of organisational discretion the ANP is afforded.

If using the seven domains of reconstruction as a predictor of role innovation, one would expect to see considerable change within each domain. The relationship between Nicholson's (1984) four key variables and the practice innovation outcome of role transition is illustrated in *Table 6.2*.

Table 6.2: Relationship between practice innovation and key variables				
Outcomes/ variables>	Role development	Personal development	Novelty	Discretion
Practice innovation	High	High	High	Low*- High#

* =Organisational discretion; # = Within-role discretion

Practice fragmentation

The third possible outcome of role transition is termed 'practice fragmentation'. This outcome replaces two of Nicholson's (1984) modes of adjustment, namely, 'absorption' and 'determination'. Neither absorption nor determination are seen to be applicable to work role transitions, which involve the development of a role which is both new to the individual and the organisation and for which there have been no previous role incumbents. Nicholson (1984) describes absorption to be the outcome of a transition in which the individual is not required to modify the parameters of the new role, but instead bears the burden of learning the skills, knowledge and behaviours required to perform in the role. However, in the case of advanced nursing practice, the role itself is new and has no established parameters in a general sense. As such, it is not possible at this stage in time for absorption to be a possible outcome.

Determination on the other hand is epitomised as being the opposite to the absorption mode of adjustment. That is to say that the incumbent of the new job is already in possession of the knowledge, skills, and abilities to be able to perform in the new role and thus is relatively unaffected by the transition but is able to adjust the parameters of the role. In the context of this study, this outcome could only be achieved if an advanced practitioner from another country, already equipped with the skills and knowledge to perform in an advanced capacity, became the incumbent of the new position in the organisation. However, few if any, nurses in the UK are in a position at this time whereby they have been shown to have acquired all of the skills, knowledge and abilities to meet the concept of 'determination' as described by Nicholson (1984). These two modes of adjustment *will* become applicable in the UK in the future (ie. when advanced practice roles have become established). However, in the context of this study, neither outcome was appropriate or likely. The evidence from this inquiry indicates, however, that a third outcome of role transition was evident, which lay between the extremes of practice replication and practice innovation, namely, 'practice fragmentation'.

Practice fragmentation occurs as a direct result of the pressures exerted by the contingent conditions of an organisation, in particular those factors relating to organisational governance, deployment and the availability of resources. This phenomenon refers to those cases where ANPs attempt to develop and implement a new role on a part-time basis, whereupon they are required to perform in a 'traditional' nursing capacity for the remainder of the rostered time. In such cases, ANPs experience both practice innovation when acting in an advanced capacity and practice replication when undertaking their traditional nursing duties. The demands and requirements of the organisation then are central in leading to a situation of practice fragmentation, which in turn can be considered to retard the rate of practice reconstruction.

Where practice fragmentation occurs, role development can be classified as 'moderate' in terms of both rate and scope. This is because while the ANP is performing new activities which require the use of new skills, behaviours and knowledge, the rate of role development and practice competency is delayed due to the requirement of having to perform in a 'traditional' nursing capacity for part of the time. Meanwhile, the 'scope' of practice can be classed as being moderate for the same reasons.

Just as there are varying degrees of role development, which are dependent upon the duration in which the ANP spends attempting to develop new roles and activities, there are corresponding degrees of personal development. As Nicholson (1984) observes, a certain amount of personal development is an inevitable consequence of role development. The evidence from this study indicates that those factors associated with personal development were seen to increase in parallel with role development. Consequently, some ANPs reported high levels of personal development while others reported moderate levels of personal development.

Likewise, the variable novelty corresponds to the amount of time in which the study participants were involved in developing the advanced practitioner role, although the ANPs whose practice reconstruction was directed toward the delivery of direct care reported higher levels of novelty. The final variable, discretion, can be seen to have remained constant across the three modes of adjustment described in this investigation. Thus, when practice fragmentation is the outcome of role transition, ANPs once again experience moderate to high degrees of discretion within their role when acting in an advanced capacity, but low levels of discretion to alter the parameters of their practice.

The relationship between Nicholson's (1984) four key variables and the 'practice fragmentation' outcome of role transition is illustrated in *Table 6.3*.

Practice fragmentation, therefore, can be seen to comprise elements of both 'practice replication' and 'practice innovation', whereby advanced practice can be perceived of as both a contingent and transient state with the ANP moving towards opposite extremes of the practice continuum as conditions encountered within the organisation dictate (*Figure 6.1*).

Table 6.3: Relationship between practice fragmentation and key variables				
Outcomes/ variables>	Role development	Personal development	Novelty	Discretion
Practice fragmenta-tion	Moderate	Moderate	Moderate	Low* - moderate/ high#
* = Organisational discretion; # = Within-role discretion				

Figure 6.1: The transient nature of advanced practice associated with the outcome of practice fragmentation

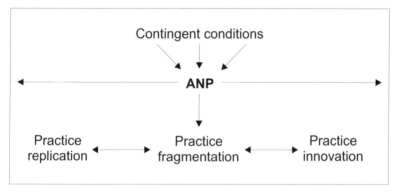

Operational outcomes of practice reconstruction — summary

It is now possible to construct a simple classification system (*Table 6.4*) to illustrate the relationship between the outcomes of practice reconstruction and Nicholson's (1984) key variables. It is also possible to account for the nature and the effect on the outcome of transition of the contingent conditions ANPs encountered during the process of practice reconstruction. It has been argued that the evidence from this study indicates that there are three possible outcomes of practice reconstruction, regardless of the direction role transition takes, namely, practice replication, practice fragmentation and practice innovation. While Nicholson's (1984) theoretical framework provided an initial basis for discussion of the data, it was necessary to adapt this model to provide a more coherent and conceptually congruent framework in which account could be taken of the transition into work roles which are both 'new' to the individual and the organisation.

Table 6.4: Matrix illusrating the relationship between the outcome of practice reconstruction and selected variables			
Outcome mode>	Practice replication	Practice fragmentation	Practice innovation
Role development	Low	Moderate	High
Personal development	Moderate	Mod<--->High	High
Novelty	Low	Moderate	High
Discretion	Mod<--->High/ Low*	Mod<--->High/ Low*	High/Low*
* = organisational discretion			

As *Table 6.4* illustrates, contingent conditions exert two effects on the nature of practice reconstruction, either impedance or facilitation. When both tendencies are present the result is compromise and practice fragmentation. It is possible that as organisational and contingent conditions are dynamic in character, in the future ANPs may move between the three outcomes of role transition. Thus while these three outcomes of practice reconstruction were observed and remained stable for the duration of this study, changing contingent conditions in the future may lead to ANPs' experiencing different outcomes at different times. In this sense advanced practice can be seen to be a highly contingent and potentially transient state. However, as stated earlier, as more ANPs enter the work force and roles become established, in principle, future versions of Nicholson's (1984) absorption and determination modes of adjustment are likely with an associated increase in stability.

Transitional outcomes of nursing studies

The operational outcomes described above vary considerably in conceptual terms from those identified in other studies of transition in advanced nurse practitioners. The main point of departure can be seen in terms of the identification of three possible outcomes of transition as opposed to a single, unifying state represented in other studies. That is to say that most studies which have explored role transition in advanced practitioners demonstrate a tendency to suggest that only a *single* outcome occurs following a linear transitional process (Anderson *et al*, 1974; Oda, 1977; Hamric and Taylor, 1989; Brown and Olshansky, 1997). Hamric and Taylor (1989) in a study of clinical nurse specialists identify this stage as *'implementation'*, whereas in a much earlier study, Anderson *et al*, (1974) proposed that nurse practitioners achieved a state of *'professional intimacy'* at completion of their training. Likewise, Oda (1977) suggested all specialist nurses achieve a state of *'role confirmation'* at the end of their transition without problem. In a more recent study, Brown and Olshansky (1997) studied the transitional process experienced by primary care nurse practitioners in the USA and concluded that over time they arrive at a stage which is termed *'broadening the perspective'*, where practitioners ultimately become effective within system. None of these studies identify that alternative outcomes are possible, only that the relevant outcome varies in terms of *when* it is achieved. As all these studies originate in North America it is possible that cultural, educational, and healthcare system differences account for their arriving at conclusions which are contrary to the findings of this inquiry. An alternative explanation of why a differentiated set of outcomes was identified in this inquiry could be related to an artefact of the duration of the study period. That is to say, that arrival at a point of practice innovation had not been identified in all cases because data collection ceased before ANPs had the opportunity to complete their transition successfully .

Other studies have adopted Benner's (1984) theoretical framework of novice to expert to explain the outcome of transition. The inconsistent way in which these criteria have been applied however, creates problems in their application to this study. In Benner's (1984) seminal work, she used the five stage criteria to identify expert ward nurses who were not advanced practitioners. On the other hand, Bass *et al* (1993) who explored the transition of novice clinical nurse specialists adapted the same criteria to explain the transition from experienced staff nurse to novice clinical nurse specialist. Shea and Selfridge-Thomas (1997) used the same principles in examining the transition of emergency nurse practitioners. In this instance they proposed practitioners moved from novice to advanced beginner in the first six months they were in post, and suggested it takes at least three years to move to a position of proficiency and expertise. The use of this theoretical framework is further complicated because of the possibility of applying Benner's (1984) criteria to individual *roles* the advanced practitioner performs.

So for example one ANP could be a 'competent' clinician, a 'novice' researcher, and 'proficient' in her educational role. Consequently, Benner's (1984) criteria were rejected as being appropriate to explain the outcome of role transition of ANPs in the UK at this time.

The operational outcomes identified by this inquiry then can be seen to provide specificity to the outcomes of role transition, which, on the whole, are generalised by other studies. While these outcomes may be indicative of current stage in development of the ANP role, or the duration of the study period, they nonetheless provide clarity of why and how the result of reconstruction occurred as it did for the ANPs who were the subject of this study.

Establishing a new professional identity

In addition to the operational outcomes of practice reconstruction described above, the findings from the study indicate that as a further outcome of role transition ANPs seek to gain recognition for their practice development. This can be considered to be the first stage in establishing a new and different professional identity from that of their nursing colleagues. It has been recognised that individuals can undergo a radical change in personal identity following a shift into a 'new' work role or situation (Van Maanen and Schein, 1979). However, the desire to change identity in the context of this study went beyond a simple change in personal identity that appears to accompany any transition (Schumacher and Meleis, 1994). More importantly, the change in professional identity has implications for the professional basis of nursing.

The results of this research reveal that it shares findings in common with other studies that have examined the identity of nurses entering advanced practice roles. It has been discovered that practitioners experience a disparity in their nursing identity which affects not only how they practice, but how they are perceived by other disciplines (Maguire *et al*, 1995). This is an important point that will be taken up later in the discussion.

In the context of this study, seeking recognition and establishing a new identity remain constant, regardless of the operational outcome of role transition the ANP achieves. Whether the outcome of practice reconstruction is replication, fragmentation or innovation, the ANPs still seek to have their new professional identity acknowledged and recognised.

The purpose of attempting to establish a new professional identity in the context of this investigation appears to be aimed not just toward enabling and empowering the ANP to become a more autonomous practitioner. It appeared that in attempting to establish a new identity the practitioner hoped to gain authority and recognition and to have greater influence on the contingent conditions which exert force over the transitional process. This included a desire to have greater control over day-to-day deployment issues and to influence the scope and boundaries of their practice. Ackerman *et al* (1996) view empowerment as central to advanced practice and suggest it is, *'...consistent with a flattened organisational structure, where the administrative hierarchy is replaced by shared governance'* (p72). That is to say that empowerment is seen as necessary to challenge the locus of control of the organisation.

The evidence from this study indicates that by intent or otherwise, ANPs not only experience the feeling of being 'different', but tacitly seek to establish to be recognised as practitioners with a unique professional identity. As a consequence of this process, it appears that all the case study ANPs experienced a loss in belonging and identity during the transitional process. This phenomenon is similar to that discovered in a study of neonatal ANPs in the UK (Dillon and George, 1997) whereby practitioners experienced a sense of isolation and felt that their professional identity was neither with the nursing profession, nor within the medical profession with whom they worked. This period accordingly has been identified as a time of uncertain professional identity where the new advanced practitioner is susceptible to role challenge from their nursing and medical colleagues (Sullivan *et al*, 1978). The data would appear to support this assertion, in that in all cases, the ANPs were challenged by both nursing and medical colleagues about the scope, purpose and authority of their new role and during the early stages of the transitional process, their ambiguous identity. During the period that this was at its most intense (ie. during the educational programme and the first 6–9 months in clinical practice post graduation), those ANPs for whom the outcome of practice was either practice replication or practice fragmentation sought to apply for new positions[1]. The main reason given for seeking alternative employment was related to being

1   Of the four case study ANPs to whom this relates: one considered application and made informal inquiries for another position; one applied for a position in another organisation but was unsuccessful following interview; one eventually was successful in securing full-time employment in a senior managerial capacity at another hospital; and the fourth eventually secured a lecturer position within a university.

unable to implement the ANP role as desired and expected due to the intervention of various contingent conditions. This is entirely consistent with advanced practitioners in other countries who cite an inability to use their practitioner skills in the practice setting as the main reason for changing jobs (Lynaugh *et al*, 1985). This would suggest that once trained, advanced practitioners experience a need to utilise and practise the skills they have developed as part of the educational preparation for the new role. At the same time however, the evidence from this study indicates that a change in identity signals disenchantment with not only the organisation, which is seen to be constraining practice development, but also with the traditional nursing role.

One way in which disenchantment with traditional nursing roles was manifest was in the way in which the case study ANPs appeared to experience a conflict in their professional identity. While, without exception, they all espoused the virtues of nursing and its under-pinning philosophy, each, perhaps to some degree unconsciously, sought to distance themselves from that traditional identity, in order to be recognised in a unique and new capacity. That is not to say that ANPs intentionally devalue nursing or nurses who continue in a more traditional role. On the contrary, their contribution was on the whole acknowledged and welcomed. It is merely that in the context of their own development, ANPs associated themselves with a different identity. The notion of practitioners submerging their nursing identity is not new. Likewise, the lack of agreement between their espoused philosophies (what they say) and the philosophies in use (what they do) has been observed elsewhere (Conway, 1996). In ANPs case studies have found that during educational preparation for advanced practice, nurses experience a temporary loss of identity, along with a loss of nursing skills, as a consequence of having to learn new skills and theory more commonly associated with the practice of medicine (Anderson *et al*, 1974; Roberts *et al*, 1997). However, while this was partly true of the nurses in this study, the desire to develop a new identity continued following the educational preparation for the advanced practitioner role. A more logical explanation for this phenomenon becomes apparent when examining the assertion that a nurse's identity,

'... *appears to be influenced by certain factors such as education, philosophy, socialization, professional relationships, and the nature of clinical practice.*' (Maguire *et al*, 1995, p54)

If this is held to be true, that ANPs seek to establish a new identity is unsurprising. For in examining each of these elements it can be seen that ANPs: undergo separate education; develop a new philosophy of how their role should be ideally enacted; undergo role socialization that results in altered professional relationships; experience substantial changes in boundaries and components of clinical practice. Moreover, this is seen to occur regardless of role orientation being directed toward the delivery of direct care or the system of care delivery. In other words, all the factors that influenced the development of their 'traditional' nursing identity are subjected to re-definition during their educational preparation and subsequent reconstruction of practice. This assertion is supported by the findings of a relatively recent US study of neonatal nurse practitioners (Beal et al, 1996) that concluded that advanced practitioners had only a very weak nursing identity due to both the way in which the role had been enacted, but also because of the role socialization processes in which practitioners engaged. Moreover, the institutional philosophy, which is conveyed via organisational governance, to some degree reinforces the notion that ANPs should no longer consider themselves to be nurses in a traditional sense. At the same time, ANPs do not consider their identity to be that of pseudo-medical practitioners, despite inevitable comparisons being made by their nursing colleagues and on occasions, the ANPs themselves. The evidence from this study clearly indicates that ANPs seek to create a new identity (Kelso and Massaro, 1994) which remains rooted within a nursing paradigm but is seen to be different from the way in which a traditional nurse is generally acknowledged and stereotyped. In some settings, such as high dependency units, this may be more difficult for advanced practitioners to achieve given the inherently medical focus of the role (Beal *et al,* 1996), especially when the orientation is directed toward the delivery of direct care or medical replacement.

The evidence from this inquiry indicates that the development of a new identity is embedded in the status afforded the practitioner while involved in clinical practice. This is manifest by the practitioner whose practice orientation is directed toward the delivery of direct care being more empowered in patient management and decision making. They have greater authority and practice independence allowing them to achieve some degree of role autonomy and discretion, which in turn are seen to be the hallmarks of professional practice (McKay, 1997). When role transition is oriented toward the system of care delivery, the development of a new nursing identity is embedded less in the acquisition of clinical skills and privileges and more in the focus of the activities in which the ANP is involved. Some authors suggest that enhancing the clinical status of advanced practice nurses by allowing them opportunities for professional growth and personal satisfaction enhances practice development and increases the effectiveness of advanced practitioners (Ventura, 1988). In the context of this discussion however, enhancing clinical status has been seen as a factor which has enables ANPs to take a step toward establishing a new professional identity.

A further reason why ANPs may seek pro-actively to alert colleagues to the establishment of a new identity, is that in some cases it is acknowledged that their role as an advanced practitioner is not particularly 'visible' in terms of both where and how they practice. This meant that just as in studies of expertise, which found difficulty in recognising expert practice that took place in low technological settings and that was of low visibility (Sutton and Smith, 1995), the advanced practitioners actively sought ways in which they could be recognised as having a different nursing identity. For example, one way in which this was achieved was to adopt the formal title of 'advanced nurse practitioner', which while not used in the public domain during contacts with patients and their relatives, was frequently used in communication and correspondence with colleagues to signal a different professional identity. Others engaged in public speaking in professional forums in order not only to disseminate the development of their role, but also to increase their visibility as 'advanced practitioners'. A legitimate question that this raises is, are these strategies simply concerned with developing personal egos or is there a more fundamental reason underlying the development of a new identity?

Arguably, the answer lies in the concepts of escapism and gaining professional power. The evidence from the study clearly indicates that in all cases, contingent conditions, dominated by organisational governance, exert influence on the process and outcome of practice reconstruction, even when the result is practice innovation. Furthermore, while ANPs experience increased degrees of practice independence and autonomy, the locus of control for role development remained with physicians and nurse administrators. In some ways therefore, advanced practitioners can be seen to have simply given up one subservient role for another with a different title. However, there are elements to the role transition that suggest that these practitioners are seeking to escape the shibboleths that have held nursing back in the past. The development of their knowledge, skill and practice base divorces their professional identity from that of traditional nurses and allows them to experience greater practice independence and to achieve recognition. In fact recognition is fundamental to the establishment of a new nursing identity and is achieved in a number of ways. Professional recognition, afforded at a national level, is evident via the acknowledgement of advanced practitioners within the clinical nursing structure. At a local level however, there were a number of other ways in which recognition was acknowledged. These included: a perceived change of status within the organisation; a change in work title; altered relationships and work practices with professional colleagues; and not least of all, increased prestige for the organisation following the practitioner's role transition.

In achieving such recognition ANPs come to be seen as experts and specialists who are called upon not only by nursing staff, but medical practitioners for advice, support and so on. At this point, the discussion concerning the development of a new professional identity for advanced nurse practitioners is analogous with Skidmore and Friend's (1984) research about the specialisation of community psychiatric nurses. Skidmore and Friend (1984) attest that practitioners who can be seen to have specialised have,

'... developed a special knowledge which excludes intrusion; it gives the practitioner security in that [s]he has developed knowledge others do not have; status, in that [s]he is often consulted by others and escapism in that, because [s]he holds this power of knowledge, [s]he can develop [her] role to suit [her]self.' (Skidmore and Friend, 1984, p203)

Thus, by escaping from a traditional nursing identity, advanced practitioners may be in a stronger position to develop their own practice and power base in healthcare delivery. When examining the development of nurse practitioners that work in primary care settings in the USA, this can be seen to have been achieved to a large degree. In the context of the UK the establishment of a separate, yet associated, identity would also serve the purposes of the UKCC and others in trying to achieve professional recognition and status for nursing. The UKCC seeks to ensure this by requiring higher level practitioners to maintain their professional 'nursing' registration in order to practice. The establishment of a separate identity, combined with practice developments that push beyond traditional boundaries, ultimately serves to legitimise nursing as a profession in its own right (Holyoake, 1996).

There are, therefore, both practical and political benefits to ANPs' developing a new professional identity, in addition to any personal status achieved. That this was a deliberate strategy on the part of the UKCC appears unlikely. Rather, it was a contrivance of circumstance and opportunity. The circumstances which acted as a catalyst to the development of the advanced practice role, such as the reduction in junior doctors' hours, has arguably allowed the UKCC to seize the opportunity to drive home its own political agenda of the professionalisation and empowerment of nursing. That the numbers of advanced practitioners at this point in time are relatively few merely represents the embryonic stage of such a strategy. It is likely that this agenda will continue to be pursued when criteria for a 'higher level of practice' are published. The danger inherent in such a strategy however is that the development of a new nursing identity will be dissociated from the practice of nursing. The evidence from this study reveals that ANPs are already having their identity associated with that of physicians rather than nurses. Furthermore, in some cases, while ANPs espouse the virtues and values of nursing, when they are required to engage in traditional nursing behaviours they appear to de-value those experiences by bemoaning the lost opportunities they have had to develop their 'new' role. This appears to be in direct contrast to the view that advanced practice nurses should value their nursing heritage (O'Flynn, 1996). The potential outcome if such a view were to become widely held is the likelihood that in attempting to achieve a new professional identity, advanced practitioners could break away from the mainstream of nursing and develop their own professional practice association. In turn, this could benefit their goal for greater empowerment within the organisation, which at the present time as a group of separate individuals they have found great difficulty in achieving. While this would arguably provide advanced practitioners with more power to control the development of their role, it could also serve to further fragment nursing and do little to establish the recognition of nursing as a major professional discipline. We will have to wait and see whether advanced and specialist practitioners try and break away from the mainstream of nursing, or whether they will embrace and value their heritage and remain within the discipline that has traditionally been recognised as nursing.

References

Ackerman M, Norsen L, Martin B *et al* (1996) Development of a model of advanced practice *Am J Crit Care* **5**(1): 68–73

Anderson E, Leonard B, Yates J (1974) Epigenesis of the nurse practitioner role *Am J Nurs* **74**(10):1812–16

Bass M, Rabbett P, Siskind M (1993) Novice CNS and role acquisition *Clin Nurs Spec* **7**(3):148–52

Beal J, Maguire D, Carr R (1996) Neonatal nurse practitioners: identity as advanced practice nurses. *J Gyn Neo Nurs* **25**(5):401–6

Benner P (1984) *From Novice to Expert.* Addison-Wesley, London

Black J, Ashford S (1995) Fitting in or making jobs fit: factors affecting mode adjustment for new hires. *Human Rel* **48**(4):421–37

Brown M, Olshansky E (1997) From limbo to legitimacy: a theoretical model of the transition to the primary care nurse practitioner role. *Nurs Res* **46**(1):46–51

Conway J (1996) *Nursing Expertise and Advanced Practice* Quay Books, Mark Allen Publishing Ltd, Dinton, Wilts

Dillon A, George S (1997) Advanced neonatal nurse practitioners in the United Kingdom: where are they and what do they do? *J Adv Nurs* **25**:257–64

Glen S, Waddington K (1998) Role transition from staff nurse to clinical nurse specialist: a case study. *J Clin Nurs* **7**:283–90

Hamric A, Taylor J (1989) Role development of the CNS. In: Hamric A, Spross J, eds. *The Clinical Nurse Specialist in Theory and Practice.2nd edition.* W B Saunders, Philadelphia: 41–82

Holyoake D (1996) Medicine is still big brother. *Nurs Stand* **10**(28):11

Kelso L, Massaro L (1994) Implementation of the acute care nurse practitioner role. *AACN Clin Issues* **5**(3):404–7

Lynaugh J, Gerrity P, Hagopian G (1985) Patterns of practice: Master's prepared nurse practitioners. *J Nurs Educ* **24**:291–5

Maguire D, Carr R, Beal J (1995) Creating a successful environment for neonatal nurse practitioners. *J Peri Neo Nurs* **9**(3): 3–61

McKay S (1997) The route to true autonomous practice for midwives. *Nurs Times* **93**(46):61–2

Nicholson N (1984) A Theory of work role transitions. *Admin Science Quart* **29**: 172–91

O'Flynn A (1996) The preparation of advanced practice nurses. *Nurs Clin North Am* **31**(3):429–38

Oda D (1977) Specialized role development: a three-phase process. *Nurs Outlook* **25** (6):374–7

Roberts S, Tabloski P, Bova C. (1997) Epigenesis of the nurse practitioner role revisited. *J Nurs Educ* **36**(2):67–73

Schumacher K, Meleis A (1994) Transitions: a central concept in nursing. *Image: J Nurs Schol* **26**(2):119–27

Shea S, Selfridge-Thomas J (1997) The ED nurse practitioner: pearls and pitfalls of role transition and development. *J Emerg Nurs* **23**(3):235–7

Skidmore D, Friend F (1984) Specialism or escapism? *Nurs Times Com Outlook* June 13, 203–5

Sullivan J, Dachelet C, Sultz H *et al* (1978) Overcoming barriers to the employment and utilization of the nurse practitioner. *Am J Public Health* **68**:1097–103

Sutton F, Smith C (1995) Advanced nursing practice: new ideas and new perspectives. *J Adv Nurs* **21**(6):1037–43

van Maanen J, Schein E (1979) Toward a theory of organisational socialization. In: Staw B, ed. *Research in organisational Behaviour, Vol 1.* JAI Press, Greenwich, CT:209–64

Ventura M (1988) Assessing the effectiveness of nurse practitioners. *Nurs Times* **84**(9):50–1

Woods L (1999) The contingent nature of advanced nursing practice. *J Adv Nurs* **30**(1):121–8

7

Will advanced nursing practice remain an enigma?

The previous chapters have explained advanced practice as an abstract model, arguing that the transition from experienced nurse to advanced practitioner involves the reconstruction of a series of personal and practice domains. Attached to each conceptual domain is a series of properties which can be used to determine the extent and nature of practice development. It is openly acknowledged that the process of role transition is highly complex and subject to a myriad of competing factors in the social environment. This will always result in advanced practice being contingent in nature (Woods, 1999), at least for the foreseeable future. Albarran and Fulbrook (1998), when examining advanced nursing practice from an historical perspective suggested that,

> '...the struggle for advanced nursing practice has been neither coherent nor deliberate, with progress being influenced by a number of internal and external forces, some of which have hampered recognition, while others have promoted the motives and wide benefits of advanced nursing practice .' (p29)

The changing nature of policy development at both professional and legislative levels means that arriving at a consensus regarding the future direction of practice development and agreement over differing levels of practice is likely to remain unresolved in the future, just as has been so in the past. It is conceivable that the UKCC's apparent U-turn with regard to advanced practice in favour of what it now terms a 'higher level of practice' (UKCC, 1998), will simply replace one set of dilemmas regarding the nature of nursing practice with another.

Earlier, it was argued that the UKCC saw the reconstruction of nursing via the development of advanced practitioners as a way to enhance the professional status of nursing. The fact that advanced practice has now been replaced by the term a higher level of practice, does little to signal a change in the UKCC's overall aim to enhance the power base of nursing in its own right. At this stage in the early evolution of the advanced practice role it is worthwhile considering if the UKCC is likely to have its goal achieved.

The drive for professional status and acknowledgement is not new. One of the prominent traits of a profession described over forty years ago, the development of systematic theory and knowledge (Greenwood, 1957), is still regarded as something nursing has yet to achieve in the eyes of other professional groups. In this sense, the generation of nursing theory that has occurred over the past thirty years has been seen largely to be born out of a professional need (McFarlane, 1976). Nursing over recent years has attempted to generate its own substantive theoretical foundation, but is generally considered to have failed in its attempt to articulate a knowledge base which it can call unique. More recently there have been calls for nursing to abandon its search for an original body of knowledge (Nolan *et al*, 1998). Correspondingly, and by coincidence, the generation of nursing theories appears to have been in abeyance while nursing considers its future.

Arguably, one strategy that appeared to be adopted in the early 1990s in an attempt to gain momentum toward achieving the goal of having nursing attain major profession status, was the move to recognising an advanced nurse practitioner role. One of the premises of this position was the hope and anticipation that advanced *practitioners* would enhance the knowledge base of nursing where *theoreticians* had failed. The inclusion of compulsory nursing theory modules in advanced practitioner programme curricula in the USA (Shah *et al*, 1993; Hravnak *et al*, 1995; King and Ackerman, 1995), and the development of similar modules in this country, such as *'knowledge development in nursing'* (Davies, 1993), serve to illustrate that the drive for the development of a unique body of knowledge is still alive. This book has attempted to explain how advanced practitioners reconstruct their practice during the transitional process. The final question to be addressed concerns the issue of whether a unique body of nursing knowledge is synthesised during, or subsequent to, the process of role transition in which ANPs engage.

In the initial phase of practice reconstruction that was the focus of this study, there was no evidence to suggest that the theoretical development of nursing knowledge has occurred. The reason for this is that just as in the general domain of nursing, where theories have been 'borrowed' from other disciplines such as psychology, sociology and anthropology (Meleis, 1985), nurses engaging in role transition to become advanced practitioners appear to adopt a similar strategy. When their orientation is as clinicians, ANPs borrow theories and knowledge from areas such as medicine, biology, and physiology. Likewise, when they are directed toward the system of care delivery they borrow educational theories and theories of change. Consequently, it is the direction of the transition which determines the origin of the disciplines from which ANPs adapt and borrow theories. Thus, contrary to some expectations, the ANPs in this study have not synthesised any new nursing knowledge, but have merely reconstructed their knowledge base from the relevant disciplines to be able to inform their practice as advanced practitioners. This indicates that ANPs are in fact utilising 'transdisciplinary knowledge' (Retsas, 1995) which, while it has historically been condemned on grounds of doing little to enhance the development of a unique body of nursing knowledge, is becoming an increasingly accepted and advocated position (Nolan *et al*, 1998).

The findings of this study, therefore, reveal that advanced practitioners are entering what Kidd and Morrison (1988) describe as the fifth period of knowledge in nursing. This is similar to the notion of transdisciplinary knowledge but to which Kidd and Morrison (1988) refer as 'constructed knowledge'. They view constructed knowledge as being based on the integration of knowledge from equally legitimate but differing origins. The UKCC seemed to have moved toward acknowledging this position when it openly stated that practitioners should have an 'eclectic knowledge base' (UKCC, 1996, p7). The evidence from this study then clearly supports that, as opposed to developing new nursing knowledge, practitioners draw on transdisciplinary knowledge in the pursuit of advanced practice. This in itself need not exclude nursing from eventually being recognised as a major profession as, arguably, it is the way in which constructed knowledge is applied in the practice of nursing that will make the theoretical base of nursing unique.

Conclusion

This book has proposed that the transition from experienced nurse to advanced nurse practitioner involves a cycle of deconstruction-reconstruction within seven distinct personal and practice domains. This transitional process entails a journey that is highly subjective and often problematic in nature. It was discovered that from the outset, the individuals' motivation for undergoing role transition and the organisations' readiness to embrace the concept of advanced practice were in a state of disequilibrium. It has been established that from an initial stage of idealism, where ANPs and key stakeholders promote the concept of advanced practice to be something that is ultimately unachievable, practitioners experience the reality shock of attempting to construct a role within an environment of competing agendas and constraints, imposed through the process of organisational governance. It has been suggested that practice reconstruction then, is contingent in nature upon key stakeholders within the organisation and a variety of factors experienced within individual practice settings. It is asserted here that it is the nature of contingent conditions that leads to practice reconstruction taking one of two fundamental directions. The first primarily involves the ANP acting as a clinician in the delivery of direct patient care, while the second sees the ANP enacting a role whose prime purpose serve to enhance the system of care delivery. The idealised eclectic role to which some individuals in the organisation aspire and to which the UKCC also originally aspired, fail to emerge as an outcome of the reconstruction of nursing at this time.

Regardless of the direction of role orientation, the outcome of the transitional process was characterised by one of three states: practice replication; practice fragmentation; and practice innovation. While individual ANPs strove to achieve the latter, contingent conditions within the practice setting acted to mediate and sanction practice development.

The transitional process was also seen to involve the ANPs in attempting to gain recognition and status within the organisation, with the aim of escaping from what in effect was fundamentally still a subservient role. In order to achieve this goal, ANPs embarked upon trying to establish their own unique professional identity within the practice setting. In so doing, it is conjectured that the development of a new identity was ultimately seen as a means to empower advanced nurse practitioners to have greater independence and influence over the matters of healthcare delivery in the institutions within which they worked. It is proposed that this strategy indirectly serves the purpose of the UKCC in progressing its own agenda to have nursing achieve greater professional status and independence. While the latter still appears to be some way off, a change in status and identity would allow ANPs to escape from the constraints associated with a traditional nursing identity and stamp their own unique individuality and authority on the practice of nursing.

The results of this study serve to illustrate that attempts to arrive at a conclusive definition of the concept of advanced practice is fraught with difficulty. The highly individual and context-bound notion of advanced practice, which is socially constructed by actors in the social setting, suggests that striving to arrive at a global definition of advanced practice is an erroneous endeavour. The evidence from this study indicates that any definition which could be universally applied would be either too specific so as to be exclusionary, or too general to be meaningful. Frost (1998) uses a nice analogy to sum up the essence of this argument when she suggests that,

'...defining advanced practice is a bit like trying to secure jelly with drawing pins. Every time you get near to succeeding, it slips away.' (p40)

This book does, therefore, not attempt to offer a conclusive definition of the concept of advanced practice. Instead, it is suggested that the use of a practitioner profile, where change in each of the seven domains of reconstruction could be demonstrated, would serve as a more useful and meaningful indicator of the attainment of an advanced level of nursing practice. For many, however, the concept of advanced or a higher level of practice will remain an enigma.

The results of this inquiry have a number of implications for practitioners, educators and policy makers alike. In particular, all parties need to be aware not only of the contingent nature of practice reconstruction, but the dichotomised nature of role orientation. Consequently, it is suggested that *prior* to employing advanced practitioners appropriate educational requirements, person specifications, and resource implications for development of the ANP role need to be considered thoroughly. Institutions also need to consider the location of the practitioner in the organisational hierarchy and develop appropriate role objectives that are realistic and framed within the constraints of the practice discipline. To allow for integration of the ANP into the clinical environment, careful thought needs to be given to the adequate dissemination of the purpose of the new role to nursing and medical colleagues. At a policy level, the results of this study suggest that if an advanced level of practice is to be officially recognised and pursued as an avenue of professional development for nurses, criteria need to be established that are cognisant of the contingent nature and individuality of practice reconstruction. The seven domains of reconstruction identified by this study could provide a basis for a general framework of this nature.

A number of issues have been identified by this inquiry which can be taken forward as a future research agenda in exploring the concept of advanced nursing practice. Firstly, having identified the seven domains of reconstruction, the development of measurement instruments to help establish the degree of change in each personal and practice domain during the transitional process could be considered. Another question that remains to be answered is: is there any relationship between the dichotomous nature of role orientation and the way in which the seven domains are reconstructed? In terms of healthcare economics, outcome indicators could be identified that would help determine the effectiveness and efficiency of the advanced practitioner role. As this study has identified a dichotomous role orientation, different outcome measures could be developed accordingly. Thus, outcomes such as patient satisfaction, length of stay, re-admission rates, auditing of clinical records, patient management protocols and the cost effectiveness of interventions, are just some examples of the type of outcomes which could be used to evaluate the ANP role. For those ANPs whose role is directed toward the system of care delivery, audit tools would need to measure the impact of the ANP role on professional colleagues and service delivery. Arguably, of these evaluative research approaches, the latter by its nature is likely to prove most challenging. Future studies may also wish to examine the relationship between organisational governance and role effectiveness. Furthermore, studies need not necessarily be confined to secondary or tertiary care settings and could be expanded to examine the ANP role in primary care. In addition, comparative studies could be conducted between nurses undertaking innovative roles who are not educated to master's degree level and those who are, to establish if there is any significant relationship between practice performance and educational preparation.

That further research is required is obviously without question as there is a need to continue to increase our understanding of the concept of advanced practice and the role of the advanced nurse practitioner. This book has hopefully provided a theoretical and practical platform from which to proceed, while acknowledging the limitations of the multiple case study design utilised in this inquiry. Any future research agenda needs to be cognisant of not only methodological problems, but also the political and professional agendas which underpin the emergence of advanced practice as a present day phenomenon in the UK. This book has provided an initial step in understanding the complex nature of role transition and the reconstruction of nursing. As with any early theoretical abstraction, the notion of reconstructing nursing should be used a basis from which to work and further develop understanding of what is a highly complex phenomenon.

The title of this final chapter asked the question, will advanced nursing practice (or its replacement, a higher level of practice) remain an enigma? In the short-term, the likely answer is yes. One only has to reflect on similar developments in North America to appreciate that debates have continued to rage for over thirty years in relation to a range of issues concerning advanced nursing practice. In the UK, we have already seen an apparent major U-turn from the

UKCC regarding attempts to define the concept of advanced practice toward a more conservative notion of *'a higher level of practice'*. The uncertainty that continues to reign over the idea of nurses developing and expanding their roles and skills has called into question how a wide range of innovative practice developments and roles is acknowledged and recognised. Nurse practitioners and clinical nurse specialists are just two occupational groups to find themselves at the centre of the profession's hesitancy about how best to proceed with these issues. The enigma of advanced practice has, therefore, affected every level of nursing hierarchy, from individual practitioner to healthcare managers right through to policy makers and professional bodies. So, will advanced practice remain an enigma into the new millennium?

References

Albarran J, Fulbrook P (1998) Advanced nursing practice: an historical perspective. In: Rolfe G, Fulbrook P, eds. *Advanced Nursing Practice.* Butterworth-Heinemann, Oxford: 11–32

Davies B (1993) An international approach to Master's-level preparation for clinical nurse specialists. *J Adv Nurs* **18**:1429–33

Frost S (1998) Perspectives on advanced practice: an educationalist's view. In: Rolfe G, Fulbrook P, eds. *Advanced Nursing Practice.* Butterworth-Heinemann, Oxford: 33–42

Greenwood E (1957) Attributes of a profession. *Social Work* **2**(3):44–5

Hravnak M, Kobert S, Risco K *et al* (1995) Acute care nurse practitioner curriculum: content and development process. *Am J Crit Care* **4** (3):179–88

Kidd P, Morrison E (1988) The progression of knowledge in nursing research: a search for meaning. *Image: J Nurs Schol* **20**(4):222–4

King K, Ackerman M (1995) An educational model for the acute care nurse practitioner. *Crit Care Nurs Clin North Am* **7**(1):1–7

McFarlane J (1976) The role of research and the development of nursing theory. *J Adv Nurs* **1**:443–51

Meleis A (1985) *Theoretical nursing: development and progress.* JB Lippincott, Philadelphia

Nolan M, Lundh U, Tishelman C (1998) Nursing's knowledge base: does it have to be unique? *Br J Nurs* **7**(5):270–76

Retsas A (1995) Knowledge and practice development: toward an ontology of nursing. *Aus J Adv Nurs* **12**(2):20–5

Shah H, Sullivan D, Lattanzio J *et al* (1993) Preparing acute care nurse practitioners at the University of Connecticut. *AACN Clin Iss* **4**(4):625–9

United Kingdom Central Council for Nursing, Midwifery and Health Visiting. (1996) *PREP - The Nature Of Advanced Practice – An Interim Report.* UKCC, London

United Kingdom Central Council for Nursing, Midwifery and Health Visiting (1998) *A Higher Level Of Practice: Consultation Document.* UKCC, London

Woods L (1999) The contingent nature of advanced nursing practice. *J Adv Nurs* **30**(1):121–8

Index

A

advanced level practice 105

advanced nurse practitioner 1–2, 25, 27, 36, 41, 42, 48, 62, 64, 83, 101, 104, 110, 116, 117, 122–3, 126

advanced practice
~ concept of 75, 126
~ definition of 1, 4, 124
~ models of 5, 8, 67

advanced practice nurses
~ clinical status 116

advanced practitioner 76

advanced practitioners
~ development of 80
~ role 108

affect 75, 78

autonomy 3, 5,115

B

behaviour 75, 78

Benner's (1984) novice-to-expert 75

C

case study 44, 49, 79, 103, 113,126

clinical credibility
~ establishment of 91

clinical judgement 3, 4, 5, 68

clinical nurse specialist 3, 6, 9, 13, 16, 63, 97, 111, 127

Code of Professional Conduct *xvii*

cognition 5, 26, 65, 67,75,78,80

collaborative relationships 13

concept of advanced practice 75

consultant nurses *xvii*, 77

critical
~ reflection 8
~ thinking 4, 8, 80

D

decision making 5

deconstruction 71

deconstruction- reconstruction cycle 69, 70–1,76, 78, 82, 123

Department of Health
~ A Vision of the Future *xiv*
~ Heathrow Debate *xiv*
~ Making a Difference *xiv*

discretion *xix*, 59, 84, 102, 103, 105

E

educational preparation *xv*, 7, 62, 87, 90, 93,114–15, 126

emergency nurse practitioner 87

exercising accountability *xvii*

expert 2, 4, 5, 23, 26, 27, 32, 80, 111, 116, 117

expertise *ix, xvii, 6,* 13, 23, 25, 27–8, 34, 95, 116,

G

grounded theory 54

H

higher level of practice *x*, 64, 75, 81, 118, 121, 125–6

I

identity 75, 78
~ nursing 114, 116
~ professional 59, 92, 101, 112, 113, 117, 118, 124